T0263807

Heart Failure in Women

Editors

GINA PRICE LUNDBERG
LAXMI S. MEHTA

HEART FAILURE CLINICS

www.heartfailure.theclinics.com

Consulting Editor
EDUARDO BOSSONE

Founding Editor
JAGAT NARULA

January 2019 • Volume 15 • Number 1

ELSEVIER

1600 John F. Kennedy Boulevard • Suite 1800 • Philadelphia, Pennsylvania, 19103-2899

http://www.theclinics.com

HEART FAILURE CLINICS Volume 15, Number 1
January 2019 ISSN 1551-7136, ISBN-13: 978-0-323-65467-8

Editor: Stacy Eastman
Developmental Editor: Laura Fisher

© **2019 Elsevier Inc. All rights reserved.**

This periodical and the individual contributions contained in it are protected under copyright by Elsevier, and the following terms and conditions apply to their use:

Photocopying

Single photocopies of single articles may be made for personal use as allowed by national copyright laws. Permission of the Publisher and payment of a fee is required for all other photocopying, including multiple or systematic copying, copying for advertising or promotional purposes, resale, and all forms of document delivery. Special rates are available for educational institutions that wish to make photocopies for non-profit educational classroom use. For information on how to seek permission visit www.elsevier.com/permissions or call: (+44) 1865 843830 (UK)/(+1) 215 239 3804 (USA).

Derivative Works

Subscribers may reproduce tables of contents or prepare lists of articles including abstracts for internal circulation within their institutions. Permission of the Publisher is required for resale or distribution outside the institution. Permission of the Publisher is required for all other derivative works, including compilations and translations (please consult www.elsevier.com/permissions).

Electronic Storage or Usage

Permission of the Publisher is required to store or use electronically any material contained in this periodical, including any article or part of an article (please consult www.elsevier.com/permissions). Except as outlined above, no part of this publication may be reproduced, stored in a retrieval system or transmitted in any form or by any means, electronic, mechanical, photocopying, recording or otherwise, without prior written permission of the Publisher.

Notice

No responsibility is assumed by the Publisher for any injury and/or damage to persons or property as a matter of products liability, negligence or otherwise, or from any use or operation of any methods, products, instructions or ideas contained in the material herein. Because of rapid advances in the medical sciences, in particular, independent verification of diagnoses and drug dosages should be made.

Although all advertising material is expected to conform to ethical (medical) standards, inclusion in this publication does not constitute a guarantee or endorsement of the quality or value of such product or of the claims made of it by its manufacturer.

Heart Failure Clinics (ISSN 1551-7136) is published quarterly by Elsevier Inc., 360 Park Avenue South, New York, NY 10010-1710. Months of publication are January, April, July, and October. Business and editorial offices: 1600 John F. Kennedy Boulevard, Suite 1800, Philadelphia, PA 19103-2899. Periodicals postage paid at New York, NY, and additional mailing offices. Subscription prices are USD 261.00 per year for US individuals, USD 501.00 per year for US institutions, USD 100.00 per year for US students and residents, USD 300.00 per year for Canadian individuals, USD 580.00 per year for Canadian institutions, USD 315.00 per year for international individuals, USD 580.00 per year for international institutions, and USD 100.00 per year for Canadian and foreign students/residents. To receive student and resident rate, orders must be accompanied by name of affiliated institution, date of term, and the *signature* of program/residency coordinator on institution letterhead. Orders will be billed at individual rate until proof of status is received. Foreign air speed delivery is included in all *Clinics* subscription prices. All prices are subject to change without notice. **POSTMASTER:** Send address changes to *Heart Failure Clinics*, Elsevier Health Sciences Division, Subscription Customer Service, 3251 Riverport Lane, Maryland Heights, MO 63043. **Customer Service: 1-800-654-2452 (US and Canada). From outside of the US and Canada, call 314-447-8871. Fax: 314-447-8029. For print support, E-mail: JournalsCustomerService-usa@elsevier.com. For online support, E-mail: JournalsOnlineSupport-usa@elsevier.com.**

Reprints. For copies of 100 or more of articles in this publication, please contact the Commercial Reprints Department, Elsevier Inc., 360 Park Avenue South, New York, NY 10010-1710. Tel.: 212-633-3874; Fax: 212-633-3820; E-mail: reprints@elsevier.com.

Heart Failure Clinics is covered in *MEDLINE/PubMed (Index Medicus)*.

Contributors

CONSULTING EDITOR

EDUARDO BOSSONE, MD, PhD, FCCP, FESC, FACC
Director, "Cava de' Tirreni" Cardiology Unit,
Heart Department, Scuola Medica Salernitana,
University Hospital, Lauro (AV), Salerno, Italy

EDITORS

GINA PRICE LUNDBERG, MD, FACC
Clinical Director, Emory Women's Heart
Center, Emory University School of Medicine,
Atlanta, Georgia, USA

LAXMI S. MEHTA, MD, FACC, FAHA
Medical Director, Heart Failure and Cardiac
Transplant, The Ohio State University,
Columbus, Ohio, USA

AUTHORS

NEELUM T. AGGARWAL, MD
Associate Professor, Department of
Neurological Sciences, Rush Alzheimer's
Disease Center, Rush University Medical
Center, Chicago, Illinois, USA

CHRISTINE M. ALBERT, MD, MPH
Professor, Department of Medicine,
Cardiology Division, Brigham and Women's
Medical Center, Boston, Massachusetts, USA

ZAKARIA ALMUWAQQAT, MD, MPH
Department of Medicine, Emory University
School of Medicine, Rollins School of Public
Health, Emory University, Atlanta, Georgia, USA

KELLY AXSOM, MD
Assistant Professor, Department of Medicine,
Division of Cardiology, Center for Advanced
Cardiac Care, Columbia University Medical
Center – NewYork-Presbyterian Hospital,
New York, New York, USA

ANA BARAC, MD, PhD
Division of Cardiology, MedStar Washington
Hospital Center, MedStar Heart and Vascular
Institute, Department of Oncology,
Georgetown University, Washington, DC, USA

LORI A. BLAUWET, MD
Associate Professor of Medicine,
Cardiovascular Medicine, Mayo Clinic,
Rochester, Minnesota, USA

WENDY BOOK, MD
Department of Internal Medicine, Division of
Cardiovascular Medicine, Emory University,
Atlanta, Georgia, USA

ELISA A. BRADLEY, MD
Department of Internal Medicine, Division of
Cardiovascular Medicine, Dorothy Davis
Heart and Lung Research Institute, The Ohio
State University, Columbus, Ohio,
USA

DANIELA R. CROUSILLAT, MD
Division of Cardiology, Harvard
Medical School, Massachusetts General
Hospital, Boston, Massachusetts,
USA

STACIE L. DAUGHERTY, MD, MSPH
University of Colorado, Aurora, Colorado,
USA

MARYJANE FARR, MD, MSc, FACC
Associate Professor of Medicine at CUMC, Medical Director, Adult Heart Transplant Program, Columbia University Medical Center – NewYork-Presbyterian Hospital, New York, New York, USA

VERONICA FRANCO, MD, MSPH
Associate Professor of Clinical Medicine, Division of Cardiovascular Disease, Co-Director, Pulmonary Hypertension Program, Advanced Heart Failure, LVAD and Transplantation Program, The Ohio State University, Columbus, Ohio, USA

MARLENA V. HABAL, MD, FRCPC
Assistant Professor, Department of Medicine, Division of Cardiology, Columbia University Medical Center – NewYork-Presbyterian Hospital, New York, New York, USA

AYESHA HASAN, MD, FACC
Professor, Clinical Internal Medicine, Director, Cardiac Transplant Program, Heart Failure Fellowship Program, The Ohio State University Wexner Medical Center, Columbus, Ohio, USA

EILEEN M. HSICH, MD
Heart and Vascular Institute, Cleveland Clinic, Cleveland Clinic Lerner College of Medicine of Case Western Reserve University, School of Medicine, Cleveland, Ohio, USA

MAYA T. IGNASZEWSKI, MD
Cooper University Hospital, Camden, New Jersey, USA

DIPTI ITCHHAPORIA, MD
Professor, Department of Medicine, Cardiology Division, Hoag Memorial Hospital, University of California, Irvine, Newport Beach, California, USA

MICHELLE M. KITTLESON, MD, PhD
Associate Professor of Medicine, Director, Education in Heart Failure and Transplantation, Director, Heart Failure Research, Smidt Heart Institute, Cedars-Sinai Medical Center, Los Angeles, California, USA

KATHRYN J. LINDLEY, MD
Assistant Professor of Medicine, Cardiovascular Division, Washington University in St. Louis, St Louis, Missouri, USA

GINA LUNDBERG, MD, FACC
Clinical Director, Emory Women's Heart Center, Emory University School of Medicine, Atlanta, Georgia, USA

NIDHI MADAN, MD, MPH
Cardiology Fellow, Department of Medicine, Cardiology Division, Rush University Medical Center, Chicago, Illinois, USA

VALLERIE V. McLAUGHLIN, MD
Kim A. Eagle MD Endowed Professor of Cardiovascular Medicine, Associate Chief, Division of Cardiovascular Medicine, Director, Pulmonary Hypertension Program, University of Michigan, Ann Arbor, Michigan, USA

LAXMI MEHTA, MD, FACC, FAHA
Medical Director, Heart Failure and Cardiac Transplant, The Ohio State University, Columbus, Ohio, USA

JANE L. MEISEL, MD
Department of Hematology and Medical Oncology, Winship Cancer Institute, Emory University School of Medicine, Atlanta, Georgia, USA

GINA MENTZER, MD
Invasive Cardiologist, Heart Failure and Transplant Specialist, Pioneer Heart Institute, Cardiovascular Clinic of Nebraska, LLC, Lincoln, Nebraska, USA

SUSMITA PARASHAR, MD, MPH, MS
Department of Cardiology, Winship Cancer Institute, Emory University School of Medicine, Atlanta, Georgia, USA

ILEANA L. PIÑA, MD, MPH
Professor of Medicine, Professor of Epidemiology and Population Health, Division of Cardiology, Montefiore Medical Center, Albert Einstein College of Medicine, Bronx, New York, USA

ANDREA M. RUSSO, MD, FHRS
Cooper University Hospital, Camden, New Jersey, USA

JOHN J. RYAN, MD
Division of Cardiovascular Medicine,
Department of Medicine, University
of Utah, Salt Lake City, Utah,
USA

ANITA SARAF, MD, PhD
Department of Internal Medicine,
Division of Cardiovascular Medicine,
Emory University, Atlanta, Georgia,
USA

ANJAN TIBREWALA, MD
Department of Internal Medicine, Division of
Cardiology, Northwestern University,
Feinberg School of Medicine, Chicago, Illinois,
USA

AMANDA K. VERMA, MD
Cardiovascular Fellow, Cardiovascular
Division, Washington University in St. Louis, St
Louis, Missouri, USA

**ANNABELLE SANTOS VOLGMAN, MD,
FACC, FAHA**
Professor, Department of Medicine,
Cardiology Division, Rush University Medical
Center, Chicago, Illinois, USA

MARY NORINE WALSH, MD, MACC
Medical Director, Heart Failure and Cardiac
Transplant, Saint Vincent Heart Center,
Indianapolis, Indiana, USA

MALISSA J. WOOD, MD
Associate Professor of Medicine, Division of
Cardiology, Harvard Medical School,
Massachusetts General Hospital, Boston,
Massachusetts, USA

CLYDE W. YANCY, MD, MSc
Department of Internal Medicine, Division of
Cardiology, Northwestern University, Feinberg
School of Medicine, Chicago, Illinois, USA

LILI ZHANG, MD, MS
Fellow, Division of Cardiology, Montefiore
Medical Center, Bronx, New York, USA

Contents

Preface: Heart Failure in Women: An Increasing Health Concern　　　　xiii

Gina Price Lundberg, Laxmi S. Mehta, and Eduardo Bossone

Sex-Specific Differences in Risk Factors for Development of Heart Failure in Women　　　1

Gina Price Lundberg, Mary Norine Walsh, and Laxmi S. Mehta

> Sex specific differences exist in the impact of risk factors for the development of heart failure (HF). Addressing these differences can have an impact on prevention of HF. This article reviews sex-specific risk factors associated with development of HF. These risk factors include current smoking, diabetes, hypertension, and myocardial infarction. Other risks for HF are toxins, inflammation, and other chronic conditions, such as sleep breathing disorders, anemia, obesity, and renal insufficiency. Some of these risks factors present risk reduction opportunities that may improve outcomes.

Heart Failure with Preserved Ejection Fraction in Women　　　9

Anjan Tibrewala and Clyde W. Yancy

> Heart failure with preserved ejection fraction (HFpEF) is an increasingly prevalent condition, particularly in women. Comorbidities, including older age, obesity, diabetes mellitus, hypertension, and hyperlipidemia, are risk factors and define phenotypic profiles of HFpEF in women. The condition has a relatively high burden of morbidity and mortality, with phenotypic profiles potentially characterizing risk of hospitalization and mortality. Based on limited data, nonpharmacologic and pharmacologic treatments may provide benefit; however, compelling evidence-based, disease-modifying treatments are needed. Many unanswered questions about HFpEF in women warrant further investigation to improve understanding of the disease and provide better patient care.

Heart Failure with Reduced Ejection Fraction in Women: Epidemiology, Outcomes, and Treatment　　　19

Gina Mentzer and Eileen M. Hsich

> There are millions of people affected by heart failure with reduced ejection fraction (HFrEF) as diagnosed with ejection fraction 40% or less by imaging. Established therapies have been proven through clinical trials on lifestyle interventions, medications, and devices for HFrEF to improve quality of life, heart function, and survival. Although there are more men than women suffering with HFrEF, there are no prospectively proven, sex-specific guideline therapies because women have been underrepresented in clinical trials. Current recommendations for medications in women with HFrEF are described in this article.

Peripartum Cardiomyopathy: Progress in Understanding the Etiology, Management, and Prognosis　　　29

Kathryn J. Lindley, Amanda K. Verma, and Lori A. Blauwet

> Occurring in approximately 1 in 1000 live births in the United States, peripartum cardiomyopathy (PPCM) is characterized by left ventricular ejection fraction reduced to less than 45% near the end of pregnancy or within the first 5 months after delivery.

Although the cause of PPCM remains unclear, increasing evidence supports a complex interaction of genetic and environmental factors contributing to angiogenic imbalance, which may lead to myocardial dysfunction in a susceptible woman. This article reviews the progress that has been made regarding understanding of the cause, management, and natural history of PPCM.

Stress-Induced Cardiomyopathy   41

Lili Zhang and Ileana L. Piña

Stress-induced cardiomyopathy is characterized by reversible myocardial injury with distinctive regional wall motion abnormalities of the left ventricle, usually precipitated by an emotional or physical stressor. This condition has a strong predilection for older women and has a trend of increasing incidence. The diagnosis can be made based on symptoms, biomarkers, electrocardiogram, coronary angiogram, and noninvasive imaging. It is frequently complicated by acute heart failure, cardiogenic shock, arrhythmias, left ventricular outflow tract obstruction, and ventricular thrombi. Evidence of the treatment of stress-induced cardiomyopathy is limited. Prognosis is not benign; it carries substantial mortality, similar to that of acute coronary syndrome.

Atrial Fibrillation and Heart Failure in Women   55

Nidhi Madan, Dipti Itchhaporia, Christine M. Albert, Neelum T. Aggarwal, and Annabelle Santos Volgman

Atrial fibrillation often occurs as a cause or consequence of heart failure. Clinical outcomes are worse when atrial fibrillation and heart failure coexist. There are important sex-related differences in the incidence, prevalence, pathophysiology, treatment, and outcomes of these patients. Women with heart failure are at greater risk of developing atrial fibrillation than men, and more women with atrial fibrillation develop heart failure. More women die of atrial fibrillation-related strokes. Despite significant morbidity and mortality, current treatments for women are inadequate. This review explores sex differences in atrial fibrillation and heart failure, emphasizing risk stratification and treatments to improve clinical outcomes.

Breast Cancer and Heart Failure   65

Zakaria Almuwaqqat, Jane L. Meisel, Ana Barac, and Susmita Parashar

Heart failure and breast cancer have shared risks and morbidities. Multimodality therapies for breast cancer, including conventional chemotherapy, targeted therapeutics, radiation therapy, and hormonal agents, may make patients more susceptible to asymptomatic left ventricular dysfunction and clinical heart failure during and after treatment. New or preexisting left ventricular dysfunction may lead to interruptions in cancer treatment and limit options of breast cancer systemic therapy, leading to adverse outcomes. Early recognition and management of cardiovascular risk factors before, during, and after cancer treatment are of utmost importance. This review presents advances, challenges, and opportunities for cardiovascular care in contemporary breast cancer treatment.

Valvular Heart Disease and Heart Failure in Women   77

Daniela R. Crousillat and Malissa J. Wood

Valvular heart disease and heart failure remain important causes of cardiovascular disease among women in the United States. Mitral regurgitation, aortic stenosis, and tricuspid regurgitation are the most common valvular lesions among men and women. This review focuses on gender differences in the epidemiology, treatment, and outcomes of mitral regurgitation, aortic stenosis, and tricuspid regurgitation. The authors also review the unique management of valvular heart disease in pregnancy.

Heart Failure in Women with Congenital Heart Disease 87

Elisa A. Bradley, Anita Saraf, and Wendy Book

Heart failure remains the most common cause of morbidity and mortality in adults with congenital heart disease (CHD). Although gender-specific outcomes are not robust, it seems that women with CHD may be more affected by late heart failure (HF) than men. A specialized and experienced adult CHD team is required to care for these women as they age, including assessment for reversible causes of HF and in the management of pregnancy, labor, and delivery.

Advanced Therapies for Advanced Heart Failure in Women 97

Marlena V. Habal, Kelly Axsom, and Maryjane Farr

Women with advanced heart failure (HF) are underrepresented in trials of short-term and durable mechanical circulatory support although they derive similar benefit. In acute HF, intensive medical and interventional therapies are effective but underutilized. The smaller, newer generation, left ventricular assist devices (LVADs) have increased the feasibility of durable support in women. Women frequently present late, with more comorbidities, emphasizing the need for timely referral. Compared with men, the stroke risk is higher in women with an LVAD. Increased representation in clinical trials and a better understanding of the psychosocial issues affecting women is essential.

Implantable Cardioverter-Defibrillators and Cardiac Resynchronization Therapy in Women 109

Maya T. Ignaszewski, Stacie L. Daugherty, and Andrea M. Russo

Implantable cardioverter-defibrillator and cardiac resynchronization therapy devices have been prescribed for patients with heart failure for several decades. Factors leading to increased usage include significant enhancements in technology and availability of multiple randomized clinical trials demonstrating their benefit with improved implementation of evidence-based guidelines. Despite these advances, gaps still exist in the utilization and referral of these devices, particularly among women. This article reviews the literature on these devices with a focus on gender differences and proposes reasons for why they exist.

Heart Transplantation in Women 127

Ayesha Hasan and Michelle M. Kittleson

Over the past 5 decades, heart transplantation has become an established therapy with greater quality of life and survival than expected from end-stage heart failure. Nonetheless, challenges still exist, especially for women undergoing heart transplantation. Women have greater post-transplant survival than their male counterparts but worse quality of life. Pregnancy may occur, especially because more women are reaching child-bearing age after transplantation. Successful outcomes have been reported but require a systematic multidisciplinary approach. Women are more likely to be sensitized, with preformed anti-human leukocyte antigens antibodies related to prior pregnancies, posing challenges for their pretransplant and post-transplant management.

Pulmonary Hypertension in Women   137

Veronica Franco, John J. Ryan, and Vallerie V. McLaughlin

Prevalence of pulmonary arterial hypertension (PAH) is higher in women, and the mechanism remains unclear. Prognosis is overall better for female compared with male patients with PAH. Pregnancy is associated with significant risk, mortality, and morbidity in patients with PAH; consensus guidelines recommend against pregnancy and counsel about early termination in these patients. Recent advances in treatment showed improvement in prognosis in small case reports of pregnant patients with PAH, particularly with the early use of parental prostacyclin. Education remains fundamental for women with PAH of childbearing age for pregnancy prevention as well as discussion about birth control methods.

HEART FAILURE CLINICS

FORTHCOMING ISSUES

April 2019
Imaging the Failing Heart
Mani A. Vannan, *Editor*

July 2019
Hormonal and Metabolic Abnormalities in Heart Failure Patients: Pathophysiological Insights and Clinical Relevance
Pasquale Perrone Filardi, *Editor*

October 2019
Hypertensive Heart Disease
George L. Bakris and Ragavendra R. Baliga, *Editors*

RECENT ISSUES

October 2018
Recent Advances in Management of Heart Failure
Ragavendra R. Baliga and Umesh C. Samal, *Editors*

July 2018
The Right Heart-Pulmonary Circulation Unit
Eduardo Bossone and Luna Gargani, *Editors*

April 2018
Clinical and Molecular Aspects of Cardiomyopathies: On the Road from Gene to Therapy
Sharlene M. Day, Perry M. Elliott, and Giuseppe Limongelli, *Editors*

SERIES OF RELATED INTEREST

Cardiology Clinics
http://www.cardiology.theclinics.com/

THE CLINICS ARE AVAILABLE ONLINE!
Access your subscription at:
www.theclinics.com

Preface

Heart Failure in Women: An Increasing Health Concern

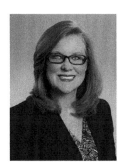 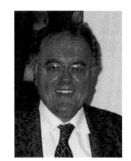 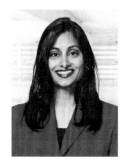

Gina Price Lundberg, MD, FACC   Eduardo Bossone, MD, PhD, FCCP, FESC, FACC   Laxmi S. Mehta, MD, FACC, FAHA

Editors

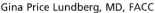

Cardiovascular disease is the number one cause of mortality in women the United States.[1] Much focus has been placed on coronary heart disease awareness, treatment, and prevention in women, yet heart failure is an equal and growing concern for morbidity and mortality among American men and women. Approximately 6.5 million US adults have heart failure, of which 3.6 million of them are women. In addition, an estimated 505,000 new cases of heart failure will occur annually in women, and the overall prevalence of heart failure among men and women continues to rise in the United States.[1]

Sex-specific differences exist in the risk factors, cause, and types of heart failure as well as the treatment and prognosis. Recognition of these sex-specific differences is necessary to advance the science and clinical care of women with heart failure. The current issue of *Heart Failure Clinics* includes thirteen sections, which review the epidemiology, cause, and prognosis of heart failure in women. Articles specific to treatment of heart failure with preserved ejection fraction and heart failure with reduced ejection fraction, advanced therapies, and heart transplant are also included. In addition, there are articles specific to entities with higher prevalence in women, such as stress-induced cardiomyopathy and pulmonary hypertension, as well as the female-only condition of peripartum cardiomyopathy. Each article highlights the data specific and unique to women.

We would like to thank the contributing authors, who are experts in cardiovascular disease and have a special interest in women's health. We extend our sincere appreciation and gratitude to each of them for their dedication and time commitent in preparing their outstanding articles for this issue of *Heart Failure Clinics*.

Gina Price Lundberg, MD, FACC
Emory Women's Heart Center
Division of Cardiology
Emory University Schoold of Medicine
137 Johnson Ferry Road, Suite 1200
Marietta, GA 30068, USA

Eduardo Bossone, MD, PhD, FCCP, FESC, FACC
Cardiology Division
"Cava de' Tirreni and Amalfi Coast" Hospital
Cardiothoracic and Vascular Department
University Hospital, Salerno, Italy

Via Pr. Amedeo, 36
Lauro, Avellino 83023, Italy

heartfailure.theclinics.com

Heart Failure Clin 15 (2019) xiii–xiv
https://doi.org/10.1016/j.hfc.2018.10.001
1551-7136/18/© 2018 Published by Elsevier Inc.

Laxmi S. Mehta, MD, FACC, FAHA
Preventative Cardiology and
Women's Cardiovascular Health
Division of Cardiology
The Ohio State University
473 West 12th Avenue
Columbus, OH 43065, USA

E-mail addresses:
Gina.Lundberg@Emory.edu (G.P. Lundberg)

ebossone@hotmail.com (E. Bossone)
Laxmi.Mehta@osumc.edu (L.S. Mehta)

REFERENCE

1. Benjamin EJ, Virani SS, Callaway CW, et al. Heart disease and stroke statistics—2018 update: a report from the American Heart Association. Circulation 2018;137(12):e67–492.

Sex-Specific Differences in Risk Factors for Development of Heart Failure in Women

Gina Lundberg, MD[a],*, Mary Norine Walsh, MD, MACC[b],
Laxmi S. Mehta, MD[c]

KEYWORDS

• Gender • Women • Heart failure • Risk factors • Hypertension • Coronary heart disease • Diabetes

KEY POINTS

• Sex-specific differences exist in the importance of risk factors for the development of heart failure (HF) and addressing such differences can have an impact on prevention of HF.
• The population-attributable risk of hypertension is higher in women.
• Diabetes is a risk factor that is associated with development of HF, particularly for women.

INTRODUCTION

Heart failure (HF) is highly prevalent within the United States (US). Approximately 6.5 million US adults aged 20 years and older have HF (2.9 million men and 3.6 million women), based on 2011 to 2014 National Health and Nutrition Examination Survey (NHANES) data.[1] The prevalence of HF in the US is expected to increase by 46% from 2012 to 2030, which will result in more than 8 million people living with HF.[2] The overall incidence of new HF cases annually in US adults older than 55 years is 1,000,000, which includes 495,000 men and 505,000 women.[3,4] According to data spanning the 1950s through the 1990s from the Framingham Heart Study (FHS), the incidence of HF has not varied significantly in men; however, it has declined by one-third in women, likely due to treatment of hypertension (HTN), a risk factor affecting HF incidence differently in women and men. During this same time period, deaths from HF declined by one-third in both men and women.[3] In older adults (>65 years of age), the incidence of HF is approximately 21 per 1000 population.[1] The risk of developing HF is 1 in 5 for both sexes and overall lifetime risk of HF at age 45 years varies from 20% to 45% depending on sex, race, and lifestyle risks.[3,5]

Sex-specific differences exist in the impact of risk factors for the development of HF. Addressing these differences can have an impact on prevention of HF. This article reviews sex-specific risk factors associated with development of HF.

RISK FACTORS FOR HEART FAILURE

One-third of the US adult population has at least 1 risk factor for developing HF.[1,6] The first NHANES Epidemiologic Follow-Up Study found several independent risk factors for HF, including male sex, physical inactivity, cigarette smoking, overweight status, HTN, diabetes mellitus (DM), valvular heart disease, and coronary heart disease (CHD).[6,7] The FHS also reported several factors associated with an elevated risk of developing HF, including HTN, left ventricular (LV) hypertrophy, CHD, DM, and

Disclosure: The authors have nothing to disclose.
[a] Emory Women's Heart Center, 137 Johnson Ferry Road, Suite 1200, Marietta, GA, 30068, USA; [b] Saint Vincent Heart Center, 10330 N Meridian Street, Indianapolis, IN 46290, USA; [c] The Ohio State University, 410 West 10th Avenue, Columbus, OH 43210, USA
* Corresponding author. Emory Women's Heart Center, 137 Johnson Ferry Road, Suite 1200, Marietta, GA 30068.
E-mail address: Gina.Lundberg@emory.edu

Heart Failure Clin 15 (2019) 1–8
https://doi.org/10.1016/j.hfc.2018.08.001
1551-7136/19/© 2018 Elsevier Inc. All rights reserved.

heartfailure.theclinics.com

valvular disease.[8,9] The incidence of HF in women was driven primarily by the risk factors of DM and HTN. Although HTN was an important risk factor for men, antecedent myocardial infarction (MI) was a more important risk for men than for women.[10] Traditional risk factors, such as HTN, CHD, DM, smoking, and obesity, accounted for 52% of the HF cases according to data from Olmsted County, Minnesota.[11] The Heart and Estrogen/Progestin Replacement Study (HERS) examined 9 potential risk factors in the development of HF from 2391 postmenopausal women with established coronary artery disease (CAD). These risk factors included atrial fibrillation (AF), current smoking, DM, HTN, left bundle branch block, LV hypertrophy, MI, obesity, and renal insufficiency. The strongest predictor of HF was DM. Additionally, this study showed the risk of HF steadily increased with a higher number of risk factors (**Fig. 1**).[11]

Lifestyle factors have been demonstrated to have a meaningful impact on the incidence of HF. The lifetime risk of developing HF for men at the age of 40 years was evaluated by the Physician's Health Study. For male physicians without HF, the incidence of subsequent HF declined for those who were never smokers, were not overweight or obese, had moderate alcohol intake, exercised frequently, ate breakfast cereal weekly, and consumed abundant fruits and vegetables. This decrease in incidence was additive for increasing numbers of these negative risk factors,

and the association remained despite antecedent MI and the presence of DM and HTN.[12]

Hypertension

HTN plays a key role in the overall burden of HF due to the high prevalence of HTN in the general population.[13] The lifetime risk of HF in people with uncontrolled HTN (blood pressure [BP] >160/90 mm Hg) is 1.6 times that of those without HTN (BP <120/90 mm Hg).[3,5] Although the prevalence of HTN is similar in both genders, women from the FHS had a 3.4-fold increased risk of HF, whereas men had a 2-fold increased risk of HF. The population-attributable risk of HTN leading to HF in women was 59% and was greater than the 39% seen in men.[8] From the NHANES data, the population-attributable risk of HF due to HTN was 10.1%.[6] These differences are due to the cohorts, as well as to the years when the studies were performed.

Diabetes Mellitus

DM is a risk factor that is associated with development of HF, particularly for women.[14] The population-attributable risk of HF due to DM was 3.1% from the NHANES data, though this was thought to be underestimated owing to the limitation of self-reporting of DM.[6] In the FHS, the population-attributable risk of DM leading to HF in women was 12% compared with 6% in men.[8] Long-term follow-up data from the FHS

Heart Failure in Women

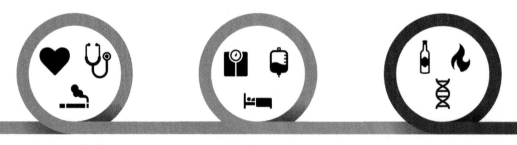

CVD Risks for HF	Conditions Associated with HF	Other Risk Factors
HTN	Obesity	Alcohol
DM	Sleep Disorder Breathing	Inflammation
CAD/MI/Ischemia	Chronic Renal Dysfunction	Genetics
Smoking	Anemia	

Fig. 1. Risk factors and associated conditions for HF in women. CAD, coronary artery disease; CVD, cardiovascular disease; DM, diabetes mellitus; HTN, hypertension; MI, myocardial infarction.

participants showed a 5-fold increased risk of HF in diabetic women, whereas diabetic men had only a 2-fold increased risk of HF.[9] A study looking at gender differences in acute HF showed that women had DM more often compared with men.[15] Additionally, early echocardiographic data from the FHS showed higher heart rates and increased evidence of LV remodeling, LV end-diastolic diameter, LV wall thickness, relative wall thickness, and LV mass corrected for height in diabetic women.[16]

Coronary Heart Disease

CHD is the most common cause of HF in the US[17]; however, it is more strongly predictive of HF in men, whereas women are more likely to develop HF in the absence of ischemia. A study looking at gender differences in acute HF showed that women had CHD less often compared with men.[15] In the FHS, the population-attributable risk of MI leading to HF in men was greater than that in women (34% vs 13%).[8] From the NHANES data on the development of HF, CHD had the greatest attributable risk, 61.6% of the cases of HF for the total population (67.9% in men and 55.9% in women).[6] More contemporary FHS data showed prior MI had a 3.5-fold and prior CHD had a 1.7-fold increased risk of HF with reduced ejection fraction (HFrEF) but no significant association seen with HF with preserved ejection fraction (HFpEF).[18] No sex-specific data are available. In a registry of hospitalized HF patients, ischemia was the principal reason for hospitalization in 15% of the patients and it was associated with an elevated risk of 60-day to 90-day mortality postdischarge.[19]

Cigarette Smoking

Limited data exist that examines cigarette smoking and incident HF. In a study looking at gender differences in acute HF, women had a history of smoking less often compared with men.[15] The NHANES showed cigarette smoking to be an independent risk factor for CHF in the US, accounting for approximately 17% of incident HF cases. Even after adjusting for CHD and other HF risk factors, there was a 45% higher risk of HF in men and 88% higher risk of HF in women who smoked.[6] More recent multivariate analyses data from the FHS showed almost 2-fold increased risk of HFpEF but no association for HFrEF.[18]

Racial and Ethnic Differences in Heart Failure

Racial differences exist in the lifetime risk for developing HF.[3] According to the Multi-Ethnic Study of Atherosclerosis (MESA) study, which included 6500 US men and women (age 45–84 years) who were free of clinical cardiovascular disease (CVD)

at baseline, the risk of developing HF is highest in African Americans, followed by Hispanics, whites, and Chinese Americans. These racial differences in risk of developing HF are likely due to difference in the prevalence of antecedent risk factors, such as HTN and DM.[3,20] Data from 156,143 postmenopausal women without HF at baseline from the Women's Health Initiative demonstrated a higher incidence of HF hospitalization in black women and lower rates in Asian or Pacific and Hispanic women compared with white women.[21] In younger participants (<50 years of age) from the coronary artery risk development in young adults (CARDIA) study, incident HF was significantly more frequent among black than white participants. Among blacks, HF occurred by age 39 years and the antecedent risk factors found were the presence of HTN, obesity, chronic kidney disease, or LV systolic dysfunction.[22]

ADDITIONAL RISK FACTORS
Alcohol

High intake and abuse of alcohol has been associated with increased risk for development of AF, MI, and HF.[23] Alcoholic cardiomyopathy (CM) results from excessive and prolonged alcohol intake and is likely linked to genetic propensity.[24] Alcoholic CM is characterized by a dilated LV, increased LV mass, and a reduced LV ejection fraction.[25] The risk of alcoholic CM increases with the quantity of alcohol intake over time. Alcohol consumption greater than 80 g per day for at least 5 years is associated with significantly increased risk.[26] There are no recent studies looking at sex-specific difference in alcoholic CM but a study from 1997 showed no differences in prevalence between men and women.[27] A study from that same time suggested that, although men may consume a higher overall amount of alcohol, women have a higher susceptibility to the toxic effects of alcohol.[28]

Inflammation

Myocarditis is a diverse group of heart-specific immune processes classified by clinical and histopathological manifestations. Myocarditis and dilated CM have a slightly greater prevalence in men than in women.[29] Up to 40% of dilated CM is associated with inflammation or viral infection.[30] Myocarditis resulting from viral infections and/or immune-mediated responses to these viruses is an important contributor to dilated CM and HF.[31] Infections from adenoviruses, echoviruses, enteroviruses, human immunodeficiency virus, and many other viruses can lead to myocarditis. Bacterial, fungal, helminthic, and protozoal infections can lead to myocarditis. Nonviral infections, such as Lyme disease, Chagas disease, and many others, can also lead to myocarditis. Exposure to these agents may lead to HF but not all patients with myocarditis develop HF. Long-term follow-up of patients with documented acute myocarditis show that only 21% of patients developed dilated CM and HF after 3 years of follow-up.[32] Men are diagnosed with myocarditis more often than women and have a worse prognosis compared with women, perhaps due to a more pronounced fibrotic response.[33]

Giant cell myocarditis (GCM) is rare and deadly, mostly affecting young to middle age adults. Early diagnosis and initiating mechanical circulatory support as a bridge to transplant is critical for survival.[34] Two studies have shown the incidence of GCM is roughly equal in men and women.[35,36] In a recent study, 13 participants were treated with modern circulatory support and 4 participants died (31%). However, the 9 participants (69%) who underwent heart transplant all survived with at least a 1-year follow-up (median follow-up was 42 months) with no recurrence of GCM.[36] A total of 20% of GCM patients have a history of other autoimmune disorders, suggesting this may be a risk factor.[30] GCM histology is characterized by the presence of giant cells, eosinophils, myocyte damage, and foci of lymphocytic myocarditis.

Myocarditis from sarcoidosis and amyloidosis are also very serious with high mortality rates. Cardiac sarcoidosis (CS) is characterized by the presence of giant cells together with granulomas and fibrosis.[37] Sarcoidosis, a multisystem granulomatous disease of unknown cause, is a worldwide disease, with a prevalence of about 4.7 to 64 in 100,000; the highest rates are reported in northern Europeans and African Americans, particularly in women.[38] CS is present in up to 25% of patients with system sarcoidosis and likely underdiagnosed. Family clustering of sarcoidosis suggests a strong genetic relationship in sarcoidosis.[39] Cardiac amyloidosis (CA) is primarily found in AL (Light-Chain) Cardiac amyloidosis (monoclonal kappa or lambda light chains) and transthyretin (TTR) amyloidosis (wild-type transthyretin).[40] In a study of 191 participants (176 men, 15 women) with histologically proven TTR CA, survival was much lower in women at 30.6 (21.1–40.1) months compared with men at 63.9 (45.8–82.0) months, suggesting the prognosis is much worse in women with CA.[40]

Genetics

Several cardiomyopathies are familial. Two well-known familial CMs are hypertrophic CM (HCM) and familial dilated CM (FDC). HCM is a CVD with autosomal dominant inheritance. Mutations in the structural and/or regulatory proteins in the sarcomere of cardiomyocytes are identified as the cause of HCM. A group of genes, including the heavy chain of beta-myosin (MYH7), myosin binding protein C (MYBPC3), cardiac troponin I (TNNI3), and cardiac troponin T (TNNT2) are frequently affected by these mutations.[41] Chromosomal point mutations in 31 autosomal chromosomes and 2 X-linked chromosomes have been linked FDC but account for only 30% to 35% of genetic causes.[42] Although genetic testing for these and other cardiomyopathies is an exciting expectation for the future, much more information about the clinical use of genotyping for cardiomyopathies is needed. Genetic testing for determination of risk of HF is not yet appropriate for clinical practice.

OTHER CONDITIONS ASSOCIATED WITH HEART FAILURE
Obesity

Obesity has an adverse impact on LV hemodynamics, cardiac structure, metabolic abnormalities, and cardiac function (systolic and diastolic).[43] Obesity[44] and overweight[6] status are risk factors for the development of both CAD and HF. The lifetime risk of HF in obese Americans (body mass index [BMI] ≥ 30 kg/m^2) is double that of those who are not obese and not overweight (BMI ≤ 25 kg/m^2).[3,5] Elevated BMI, regardless of gender, was associated with a higher risk of developing HF in the FHS, and this was not specific to only those with extreme obesity. Compared with normal BMI women, there was a 50% greater risk of developing HF in overweight women and doubling of HF risk in obese women, whereas in men there was a nonsignificant 20% increase in HF risk and 90% increase in HF risk in obese men compared with normal BMI men. In participants with HTN, there was a decreased effect of BMI on risk of developing HF compared with those without HTN.[44] Recent data from Sweden showed increased risk of HF later in life in obese young to middle-age women (ages 26–65 years), even when adjusting for baseline confounders. However, there was no association between obesity and HF in older women (>65 years of age) and development of obesity.[45] Additionally, studies have shown the so-called obesity paradox exists in HF, such that patients with higher BMI have had improved HF outcomes compared with normal BMI patients with HF, including in women.[43,46,47] In the Women's Health Study, obesity along with HTN, smoking, and DM accounted for most of the population risk of HF in women with AF.[48]

Sleep Apnea and Sleep Disordered Breathing

The 2 major types of sleep disordered breathing (SDB) are central sleep apnea (CSA) and obstructive sleep apnea (OSA) are both associated with HF.

Table 1
Heart failure risk factors, types of myocarditis, and associated conditions with sex-specific data and risk reduction opportunities

		Sex-Specific Data	Risk Reduction Opportunities
Traditional CVD Risk			
HTN		↑ significance in women	HTN control
DM		↑ significance in women	DM control
CHD		↓ incidence in women	CHD risk reduction
Tobacco or smoking		↓ incidence in women	Smoking cessation
Nonischemic CM			
Alcoholic CM		More toxic in women More common in men	Limit alcohol consumption
Myocarditis	Inflammation	↑ incidence in men	Appropriate early
	Infection	↑ incidence in men	diagnosis and
	Giant cell	Equal incidence in men and women	aggressive treatment
	CS	↑ incidence in women	
	CA	Worse prognosis in women	
Associated conditions			
Obesity		↑ incidence in women	Weight control
SDB		Women with snoring & daytime sleepiness more likely to develop HF	Sleep assessment
Renal dysfunction		↓ incidence in women	CVD risk reduction
Anemia		↑ incidence in women	Routine assessment

Abbreviations: CA, cardiac amyloidosis; CHD, Coronary heart disease; CM, cardiomyopathy; CS, cardiac sarcoidosis; CVD, cardiovascular disease; DM, diabetes mellitus; HTN, Hyper tension; SDB, sleep disorder breathing; arrow up, increased; arrow down, decreased.

CSA is associated with adrenergic activation and potentially life-threatening arrhythmias, and is independently associated with a worse prognosis in HF. OSA is also an independent risk factor for HF and has higher risk for men than women.[49] SDB is common and highly prevalent in chronic HF, acute HF, HFpEF, and HFrEF.[50] Evidence supports a causal association of sleep apnea with the incidence and morbidity of HTN, CHD, arrhythmia, HF, and stroke.[51] The 2017 American College of Cardiology (ACC), American Heart Association (AHA) and Heart Failure Society of America (HFSA) Focused Update of the 2013 Guidelines for the Management of Heart Failure[52] recommends a formal sleep evaluation for patients with symptomatic HF if there is a suspicion of SDB or excess daytime somnolence (class IIa recommendation). Women with the combination of snoring and excessive daytime sleepiness had a twofold increase in the risk of incident HF.[53] There is lack of beneficial evidence to support treatment of SDB.[54] Therefore, although SDB is a risk factor, it is not a target for treatment.

Renal Dysfunction

Deterioration of renal function can be both a consequence and a contributor to decompensated HF. HTN, DM, and other comorbidities lead to target organ damage for both the heart and the kidneys. Several epidemiologic studies have shown an independent link between risk for HF and biomarkers of renal function, such as creatinine, phosphorus, urinary albumin, or albumin-creatinine ratio.[22] A study looking at gender differences in acute HF showed women had renal failure less often compared with men.[15] The Acute Decompensated HEart Failure National REgistry (ADHERE) was a large observational study of participants hospitalized with acute decompensated HF. This study showed greater degrees of renal dysfunction in women and older participants, as well as worse in-hospital outcomes in those with renal dysfunction at the time of hospitalization.[55]

Anemia

The World Health Organization defines anemia as a hemoglobin level of less than 12 g/dL in women. Anemia is a common finding in all patients with chronic HF but is more common in women.[56] The prevalence of anemia among patients with HF seems to increase with HF severity and is found in women with both HFrEF and HFpEF. Unfortunately, patients with anemia have higher mortality compared with patients without anemia.[56] A study addressing sex differences in acute HF showed women have more anemia compared with men.[15]

RISK REDUCTION OPPORTUNITIES

The AHA Life's Simple 7 (LS7) metrics have reported a lower risk of HF with increased implementation of these metrics regardless of race or ethnicity.[57] The LS7 metrics are smoking, physical activity, BMI, diet, BP, total cholesterol, and blood glucose. In the MESA study, the group with the optimal LS7 scores had the lowest incidence of HF compared with the groups with less adherence to the LS7 metrics.[57] During the 12 years of follow-up, 4% of incident HF was reported. HF was most common in older participants, men, and black participants, which are factors that do not change with lifestyle interventions. Of the LS7 lifestyle interventions, higher baseline BP and blood glucose were statistically significant for future HF. **Table 1** outlines the risk factors for HF, types of cardiac myocarditis, and conditions associated with HF, with sex-specific data and opportunities of risk reduction and improved prognosis.

The recent ACC Foundation/AHA/HFSA guideline for the management of HF recommends that all patients at risk for HF have counseling to encourage smoking cessation; to encourage regular exercise and a healthy diet to maintain normal BMI; to discourage alcohol and drug abuse; and to control DM, lipids, BP, and metabolic syndrome risks factors.[52,58] Also included in these guidelines is the recommendation that all patients with a family history of CM and patients receiving cardiotoxins for cancer treatment maintain these lifestyle and therapy goals to prevent HF.

SUMMARY

HF is a public health burden that has a significant impact on the quality of life, life expectancy of women and men, and has a heavy economic burden. Several risk factors and chronic conditions are associated with the development of HF. Some of these are demonstrated to have sex-specific differences. Clearly preventative strategies, such as HTN and DM control, smoking cessation, optimal weight, and physical activity can be beneficial in reducing CVD and HF. Advancements in the treatment of ischemic heart disease, both acute and chronic, may help reduce the incidence of new HF cases. Also, it is necessary to underscore the importance of smoking cessation within the general population to not only reduce risks of cancer and CAD but also to reduce HF.

Given these findings, aggressive measures to reduce CHD and CVD risk factors are mandatory to make meaningful reductions on the burden of HF in the US.

REFERENCES

1. Kovell LC, Juraschek SP, Russell SD. Stage A Heart Failure Is Not Adequately Recognized in US Adults: Analysis of the National Health and Nutrition Examination Surveys, 2007–2010. PLoS One 2015;10(7): e0132228.
2. Heidenreich PA, Albert NM, Allen LA, et al. Forecasting the impact of heart failure in the United States: a policy statement from the American Heart Association. Circ Heart Fail 2013;6(3):606–19.
3. Benjamin EJ, Virani SS, Callaway CW, et al. Heart Disease and Stroke Statistics-2018 Update: A Report From the American Heart Association. Circulation 2018;1137(12):e67–492.
4. Levy D, Kenchaiah S, Larson MG, et al. Long-term trends in the incidence of and survival with heart failure. N Engl J Med 2002;347(18):1397–402.
5. Huffman MD, Berry JD, Ning H, et al. Lifetime risk for heart failure among white and black Americans: cardiovascular lifetime risk pooling project. J Am Coll Cardiol 2013;61(14):1510–7.
6. He J, Ogden LG, Bazzano LA, et al. Risk factors for congestive heart failure in US men and women: NHANES I epidemiologic follow-up study. Arch Intern Med 2001;161(7):996–1002.
7. Kannel WB, D'Agostino RB, Silbershatz H, et al. Profile for estimating risk of heart failure. Arch Intern Med 1999;159(11):1197–204.
8. Levy D, Larson MG, Vasan RS, et al. The progression from hypertension to congestive heart failure. JAMA 1996;275(20):1557–62.
9. Kannel WB, Hjortland M, Castelli WP. Role of diabetes in congestive heart failure: the Framingham study. Am J Cardiol 1974;34(1):29–34.
10. Bibbins-Domingo K, Lin F, Vittinghoff E, et al. Predictors of heart failure among women with coronary disease. Circulation 2004;110(11):1424–30.
11. Dunlay SM, Weston SA, Jacobsen SJ, et al. Risk factors for heart failure: a population-based case-control study. Am J Med 2009;122(11):1023–8.
12. Djoussé L, Driver JA, Gaziano J. Relation between modifiable lifestyle factors and lifetime risk of heart failure. JAMA 2009;302(4):394–400.
13. Wenger NK, Arnold A, Bairey Merz CN, et al. Hypertension across a woman's life cycle. J Am Coll Cardiol 2018;71(16):1797–813.
14. Kenchaiah S, Vasan RS. Heart failure in women–Insights from the Framingham Heart Study. Cardiovasc Drugs Ther 2015;29(4):377–90.
15. Nieminen MS, Harjola VP, Hochadel M, et al. Gender related differences in patients presenting with acute

heart failure. Results from EuroHeart Failure Survey II. Eur J Heart Fail 2008;10(2):140–8.

16. Galderisi M, Anderson KM, Wilson PW, et al. Echocardiographic evidence for the existence of a distinct diabetic cardiomyopathy (the Framingham Heart Study). Am J Cardiol 1991;68(1):85–9.

17. Gheorghiade M, Bonow RO. Chronic heart failure in the United States: a manifestation of coronary artery disease. Circulation 1998;97(3):282–9.

18. Ho JE, Lyass A, Lee DS, et al. Predictors of new-onset heart failure: differences in preserved versus reduced ejection fraction. Circ Heart Fail 2013; 6(2):279–86.

19. Fonarow GC, Abraham WT, Albert NM, et al. Factors identified as precipitating hospital admissions for heart failure and clinical outcomes: findings from OPTIMIZE-HF. Arch Intern Med 2008;168(8):847–54.

20. Bahrami H, Kronmal R, Bluemke DA, et al. Differences in the incidence of congestive heart failure by ethnicity: the multi-ethnic study of atherosclerosis. Arch Intern Med 2008;168(19):2138–45.

21. Eaton CB, Abdulbaki AM, Margolis KL, et al. Racial and ethnic differences in incident hospitalized heart failure in postmenopausal women: the Women's Health Initiative. Circulation 2012;126(6):688–96.

22. Bibbins-Domingo K, Pletcher MJ, Lin F, et al. Racial differences in incident heart failure among young adults. N Engl J Med 2009;360(12):1179–90.

23. Whitman IR, Agarwal V, Nah G, et al. Alcohol abuse and cardiac disease. J Am Coll Cardiol 2017;69(1): 13–24.

24. Fernandez-Sola J, Nicolas JM, Oriola J, et al. Angiotensin-converting enzyme gene polymorphism is associated with vulnerability to alcoholic cardiomyopathy. Ann Intern Med 2002;137(5 Part 1):321–6.

25. Piano MR. Alcoholic cardiomyopathy: incidence, clinical characteristics, and pathophysiology. Chest 2002;121(5):1638–50.

26. Mirijello A, Tarli C, Vassallo GA, et al. Alcoholic cardiomyopathy: what is known and what is not known. Eur J Intern Med 2017;43:1–5.

27. Fernandez-Sola J, Estruch R, Nicolas JM, et al. Comparison of alcoholic cardiomyopathy in women versus men. Am J Cardiol 1997;80(4):481–5.

28. Addolorato G, Capristo E, Caputo F, et al. Nutritional status and body fluid distribution in chronic alcoholics compared with controls. Alcohol Clin Exp Res 1999;23(7):1232–7.

29. Fairweather D, Cooper LT Jr, Blauwet LA. Sex and gender differences in myocarditis and dilated cardiomyopathy. Curr Probl Cardiol 2013;38(1):7–46.

30. Heymans S, Eriksson U, Lehtonen J, et al. The quest for new approaches in myocarditis and inflammatory cardiomyopathy. J Am Coll Cardiol 2016;68(21): 2348–64.

31. Kindermann I, Barth C, Mahfoud F, et al. Update on myocarditis. J Am Coll Cardiol 2012;59(9):779–92.

32. D'Ambrosio A, Patti G, Manzoli A, et al. The fate of acute myocarditis between spontaneous improvement and evolution to dilated cardiomyopathy: a review. Heart 2001;85(5):499–504.

33. Cocker MS, Abdel-Aty H, Strohm O, et al. Age and gender effects on the extent of myocardial involvement in acute myocarditis: a cardiovascular magnetic resonance study. Heart 2009;95(23):1925–30.

34. Ammirati E, Camici PG. Still poor prognosis for patients with giant cell myocarditis in the era of temporary mechanical circulatory supports. Int J Cardiol 2018;253:122–3.

35. Maleszewski JJ, Orellana VM, Hodge DO, et al. Long-term risk of recurrence, morbidity and mortality in giant cell myocarditis. Am J Cardiol 2015;115(12):1733–8.

36. Montero S, Aissaoui N, Tadie JM, et al. Fulminant giant-cell myocarditis on mechanical circulatory support: management and outcomes of a French multicentre cohort. Int J Cardiol 2018;253:105–12.

37. Okura Y, Dec GW, Hare JM, et al. A clinical and histopathologic comparison of cardiac sarcoidosis and idiopathic giant cell myocarditis. J Am Coll Cardiol 2003;41(2):322–9.

38. Hillerdal G, Nou E, Osterman K, et al. Sarcoidosis: epidemiology and prognosis. A 15-year European study. Am Rev Respir Dis 1984;130(1):29–32.

39. Rybicki BA, Iannuzzi MC, Frederick MM, et al. Familial aggregation of sarcoidosis. A case-control etiologic study of sarcoidosis (ACCESS). Am J Respir Crit Care Med 2001;164(11):2085–91.

40. Ronsyn M, Shivalkar B, Vrints CJ. Cardiac amyloidosis in full glory. Heart 2011;97(9):720.

41. Curila K, Benesova L, Penicka M, et al. Spectrum and clinical manifestations of mutations in genes responsible for hypertrophic cardiomyopathy. Acta Cardiol 2012;67(1):23–9.

42. Hershberger RE, Siegfried JD. Update 2011: clinical and genetic issues in familial dilated cardiomyopathy. J Am Coll Cardiol 2011;57(16):1641–9.

43. Lavie CJ, Alpert MA, Arena R, et al. Impact of obesity and the obesity paradox on prevalence and prognosis in heart failure. JACC Heart Fail 2013;1(2):93–102.

44. Kenchaiah S, Evans JC, Levy D, et al. Obesity and the risk of heart failure. N Engl J Med 2002;347(5): 305–13.

45. Halldin AK, Schaufelberger M, Lernfelt B, et al. Obesity in middle age increases risk of later heart failure in women-results from the prospective population study of women and H70 Studies in Gothenburg, Sweden. J Card Fail 2017;23(5):363–9.

46. Clark AL, Chyu J, Horwich TB. The obesity paradox in men versus women with systolic heart failure. Am J Cardiol 2012;110(1):77–82.

47. Vest AR, Wu Y, Hachamovitch R, et al. The heart failure overweight/obesity survival paradox: the missing sex link. JACC Heart Fail 2015;3(11):917–26.

48. Chatterjee NA, Chae CU, Kim E, et al. Modifiable risk factors for incident heart failure in atrial fibrillation. JACC Heart Fail 2017;5(8):552–60.

49. Gottlieb DJ, Yenokyan G, Newman AB, et al. Prospective study of obstructive sleep apnea and incident coronary heart disease and heart failure: the sleep heart health study. Circulation 2010;122(4): 352–60.

50. Cowie MR, Gallagher AM. Sleep disordered breathing and heart failure: what does the future hold? JACC Heart Fail 2017;5(10):715–23.

51. Javaheri S, Barbe F, Campos-Rodriguez F, et al. Sleep apnea: types, mechanisms, and clinical cardiovascular consequences. J Am Coll Cardiol 2017;69(7):841–58.

52. Yancy CW, Jessup M, Bozkurt B, et al. 2017 ACC/ AHA/HFSA focused update of the 2013 ACCF/AHA guideline for the management of heart failure: a report of the American College of Cardiology/American Heart Association Task Force on Clinical Practice Guidelines and the Heart Failure Society of America. J Am Coll Cardiol 2017;70(6):776–803.

53. Ljunggren M, Byberg L, Theorell-Haglow J, et al. Increased risk of heart failure in women with symptoms of sleep-disordered breathing. Sleep Med 2016;17:32–7.

54. Cowie MR. Sleep apnea: state of the art. Trends Cardiovasc Med 2017;27(4):280–9.

55. Heywood JT, Fonarow GC, Costanzo MR, et al. High prevalence of renal dysfunction and its impact on outcome in 118,465 patients hospitalized with acute decompensated heart failure: a report from the ADHERE database. J Card Fail 2007;13(6): 422–30.

56. Groenveld HF, Januzzi JL, Damman K, et al. Anemia and mortality in heart failure patients a systematic review and meta-analysis. J Am Coll Cardiol 2008; 52(10):818–27.

57. Ogunmoroti O, Oni E, Michos ED, et al. Life's Simple 7 and Incident Heart Failure: The Multi-Ethnic Study of Atherosclerosis. J Am Heart Assoc 2017;6(6) [pii: e005180].

58. Yancy CW, Jessup M, Bozkurt B, et al. 2013 ACCF/ AHA guideline for the management of heart failure: a report of the American College of Cardiology Foundation/American Heart Association Task Force on Practice Guidelines. J Am Coll Cardiol 2013; 62(16):e147–239.

Heart Failure with Preserved Ejection Fraction in Women

Anjan Tibrewala, MD, Clyde W. Yancy, MD, MSc*

KEYWORDS

- Heart failure with preserved ejection fraction • Diastolic heart failure • Sex differences • Women

KEY POINTS

- Heart failure with preserved ejection fraction (HFpEF) is the most common subtype of heart failure in women, with higher prevalence than in men.
- Several comorbidities, such as older age, obesity, diabetes mellitus, hypertension, and hyperlipidemia, define phenotypic profiles associated with HFpEF.
- Women with HFpEF are at risk of frequent hospitalization and relatively high mortality rates.
- Certain nonpharmacologic and pharmacologic interventions may provide benefit in women with HFpEF based on limited data.
- Further investigation is needed to better understand mechanisms of disease and develop therapies for HFpEF in women.

EPIDEMIOLOGY

Prevalence and Incidence

Heart failure (HF) has a substantial burden of disease in the United States. Approximately 6.5 million people age 20 years and older have HF, with about 960,000 incident cases annually.[1] HF with preserved ejection fraction (HFpEF), defined as left ventricular (LV) ejection fraction (EF) greater than or equal to 50%, has a prevalence of 36% to 59% of HF cases. An estimated 1.14% to 5.5% of the overall population have HFpEF. Variation largely depends on study periods and age distributions of studied populations.[2–4]

HFpEF is being recognized as a prevalent disease in women. An American Heart Association (AHA) Get with the Guidelines (GWTG) study indicated 63% of HFpEF cases occur in women compared with 47% of HF with mildly reduced EF cases and 36% of HF with reduced EF (HFrEF) cases (**Fig. 1**).[2] In addition, HFpEF accounts for 48% of incident HF cases, with similar rates in women and men.[5] Based on these data, it is important to recognize that (1) HFpEF is more prevalent in women compared with men, (2) incidence rates of HFpEF are similar between sexes, and (3) HFpEF is the most common subtype of HF in women.

Age

Age is a nonmodifiable risk factor associated with HFpEF in women. Older women have increasing prevalence and incidence of HFpEF.[5–7] An analysis from the Women's Health Initiative (WHI) cohort with 42,170 women showed more HFpEF hospitalizations for increasing age 60 to 69 years (hazard ratio [HR] 2.46, 95% CI 1.95–3.10) and 70 to 79 years (HR 5.22, 95% CI 4.05–6.73) relative

Disclosure Statement: The authors have nothing to disclose.
Department of Internal Medicine, Division of Cardiology, Northwestern University, Feinberg School of Medicine, Chicago, IL, USA
* Corresponding author. Northwestern University, Arkes Family Pavilion Suite 600, 676 North Saint Clair Street, Chicago, IL 60661.
E-mail address: cyancy@nm.org
Heart Failure Clin 15 (2019) 9–18
https://doi.org/10.1016/j.hfc.2018.08.002

1551-7136/19/© 2018 Elsevier Inc. All rights reserved.

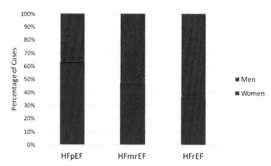

Fig. 1. Sex distribution in cases of HFpEF, mildly reduced ejection fraction (HFmrEF), and HFrEF based on data from the GWTG study. Results demonstrate that patients with HFpEF are more likely to be women compared with men. (*Data from* Steinberg BA, Zhao X, Heidenreich PA, et al. Trends in patients hospitalized with heart failure and preserved left ventricular ejection fraction: prevalence, therapies, and outcomes. Circulation 2012;126(1):65–75.)

to 50 to 59 years.[6] Furthermore, the lifetime risk for incident HFpEF in women is 10.7% at index age 45 years compared with 10.3% at index age 75 years, which suggests an equilibrium between increasing incidence of HFpEF and competing risk of mortality in older women.[7]

Alterations in ventricular-vascular stiffness underlie HFpEF in women.[8] Increased LV wall thickness (ie, LV hypertrophy) and smaller LV cavity size occur as individuals age, with more pronounced effects in women.[9,10] These anatomic changes predispose women to diastolic dysfunction. An analysis from the Prospective Comparison of ARNi [angiotensin receptor-neprilysin inhibitor] and ARB [angiotensin receptor blocker] and on Management of Heart Failure with Preserved Ejection Fraction (PARAMOUNT) trial demonstrated older women have worse LV relaxation, increased filling pressures, and increased ventricular stiffness relative to men.[10] Furthermore, aging women have increased rates of vascular stiffness, which leads to arterial hypertension (HTN), endothelial dysfunction, and microvascular disease.[11] These are all factors that contribute to the development of HFpEF.

Race

The role of race in women at risk for HFpEF is not as well studied, though may also have an impact. Black individuals are reported to have a lifetime risk of incident HFpEF of 7.7% compared with 11.2% for non-black individuals at index age 45 years.[7] Notably, this analysis is not further stratified based on sex. In the WHI cohort, hospitalization due to HFpEF was lower for black (HR 0.59, 95% CI 0.47–0.75) and Hispanic (HR 0.47, 95%

CI 0.32–0.69) women relative to white women.[6] Given that black and Hispanic individuals are more likely to have associated comorbidities, HFpEF may be underdiagnosed based on B-type natriuretic peptide (BNP) levels in these populations. Patients with African ancestry inherently have lower BNP values.[12] Additionally, black and Hispanic patients tend to be more obese, which is also associated with lower BNP values.[1] Therefore, the role of race in HFpEF remains unclear and justifies the need for further evaluation.

Comorbidities

Several chronic conditions have been associated with HFpEF (**Box 1**). Women with HFpEF have more comorbidities compared with those with HFrEF (mean 4.4 vs 3.6, $P = <.001$) with greater than 60% having at least 4 comorbidities.[13] Despite substantive data about risk factors for HFpEF, limited evidence exists specifically in women. Obesity, HTN, diabetes mellitus (DM), atrial fibrillation (AF), coronary heart disease, anemia, chronic obstructive pulmonary disease (COPD), renal dysfunction, and history of radiation are important considerations in HFpEF for all persons and perhaps especially so in women.[6,8,14]

In the WHI cohort, higher body mass index (BMI) was associated with increased risk of incident HFpEF in women in a dose-response fashion.[6] Moreover, HTN (HR 1.57, 95% CI 1.33–1.86), DM (HR 1.84, 95% CI 1.41–2.39), and AF (HR 1.39,

---

Box 1
Risk factors associated with heart failure with preserved ejection fraction in women

Demographics
- Older age
- White race

Cardiovascular risk factors
- Obesity
- HTN
- Diabetes mellitus
- Atrial fibrillation
- Coronary heart disease

Noncardiovascular risk factors
- Anemia
- Chronic lung disease
- Renal dysfunction
- History of radiation
- Lesser exposure to estrogen

95% CI 1.02–1.90) were significantly associated with increased risk of HFpEF.[6] Although history of myocardial infarction (MI) was not significantly associated with incident HFpEF, history of coronary heart disease other than MI and interim MI were associated.[6] In the Multi-Ethnic Study of Atherosclerosis (MESA) cohort, coronary artery calcium score was associated with increased incident HFpEF in women, reinforcing coronary heart disease as a risk factor.[15] In the WHI cohort, anemia was also associated with HFpEF.[6] That same analysis determined obesity and HTN were associated with two-thirds of the population-attributable risk for HFpEF in women, whereas DM and coronary heart disease made up one-fourth of the population-attributable risk.[6]

Other studies with men and women have suggested additional risks factors such as COPD and renal dysfunction exist for incident HFpEF.[8,16] Interestingly, chronic lung disease was not significantly associated with incident HFpEF in the WHI cohort, whereas renal dysfunction was not evaluated.[6] Therefore, further investigation is needed to elucidate the role of these risk factors specifically in women.

Women with a history of breast cancer who have undergone radiation therapy are at increased risk of HFpEF. A case-control study demonstrated increased risk of incident HF for higher mean cardiac radiation dose when adjusted for age, coronary heart disease, AF, and cancer stage. Among HF subtypes, increased risk of HFpEF was the primary concern rather than risk of HFrEF.[14]

Mechanistically, comorbidities such as obesity, DM, COPD, HTN, and renal dysfunction are associated with a systemic inflammatory state, which in turn leads to coronary microvascular dysfunction.[17,18] Cardiac radiation exposure is also associated with coronary microvascular disease.[14] Resultant myocyte dysfunction and interstitial fibrosis contribute to LV stiffness and diastolic dysfunction.[17]

Other mechanisms contributing to HFpEF include loss of atrial contraction and atrial-ventricular dyssynchrony in AF.[8] Furthermore, renal dysfunction predisposes individuals to sodium retention and volume expansion, which contribute to symptoms and signs of HFpEF.[8,18]

Reproductive Factors

Sex hormones are often suggested to affect a woman's cardiovascular health. In particular, menstrual cycling and pregnancy may relate to the risk of HFpEF.[19–21] Longer duration of exposure to estrogen has been thought to have cardioprotective benefits as HFpEF may develop more commonly in older women partially due to their postmenopausal status.[21] Additionally, early menopause occurring at younger than 45 years has a significantly increased risk of incident HF (HR 1.66, 95% CI 1.01–2.73).[22]

However, an analysis of reproductive features using the WHI cohort showed each year of reproductive duration (ie, older age at onset of menopause), and hence longer exposure to estrogen, did not reduce the risk of incident HFpEF. In addition, nulliparity had a higher risk of incident HFpEF, which maintained significance after adjusting for infertility.[19] Theoretically, nulliparity also increases exposure to endogenous sex hormones uninterrupted by pregnancy. This finding may be explained by an association between nulliparity and other cardiovascular risk factors unaccounted for in the analysis. Having more pregnancies, which would reduce exposure to endogenous sex hormones, was not associated with increased HFpEF.[19] Furthermore, use of estrogen-based and/or progesterone-based hormone therapy in postmenopausal women does not reduce risk of incident HFpEF.[6]

Mechanistically, estrogen has been linked to important pathways related to HFpEF. Estrogen receptors are located on the myocardium and vascular endothelium, smooth muscle cells, and adventitial cells.[11] Estrogen has been shown to modulate the renin-angiotensin-aldosterone, the nitric oxide synthase, and the natriuretic peptide systems, thereby limiting myocardial remodeling and fibrosis, promoting fluid and electrolyte homeostasis, and attenuating microvascular dysfunction. Postmenopausal women theoretically lose cardioprotective benefits via loss of estrogen stimulation in these pathways.[20,21] Overall, reproductive factors may influence HFpEF, though the current literature has mixed results and specific effects need to be elucidated.

Phenotypes of Heart Failure with Preserved Ejection Fraction

Compared with HFrEF, HFpEF seems to be more heterogeneous, having several phenotypes based on multiple contributing factors, including sex differences. However, common underlying mechanisms may suggest a degree of homogeneity.[8] Machine learning with model-based clustering has been used to identify 3 common phenotypes of HFpEF. Among these, a cardiometabolic phenotype of HFpEF was identified, with the group having 68% women, 70% obese, 52% with DM, 90% with HTN, and 62% with hyperlipidemia.[23] In a different study, 6 phenotypes of HFpEF were identified using latent class analysis. Again, a similar subgroup was present with 59% women, 100% with DM, 75% with BMI greater than 30 kg/m^2, 84% with hyperlipidemia, and median systolic blood pressure of 136 mm Hg.[24] The common factors defining a cardiometabolic profile among these studies included women with DM, obesity, HTN, and hyperlipidemia (**Fig. 2**). In addition, both studies identified a cardiorenal subgroup of HFpEF made up of older individuals who were predominantly women with low estimated glomerular filtration rates.[23,24]

Interestingly, sex was an important component in one of these analyses. For example, 2 of the 6 subgroups were made up of 100% and 96% women, whereas 2 other subgroups had 100% men.[24] This finding reinforces the notion that sex differences are important in HFpEF, with potentially unique risk factors, pathogenesis, and phenotypes in women that need to be more precisely defined.

OUTCOMES
Quality of Life

HFpEF poses a significant physical and emotional burden on par with other cardiovascular diseases. Individuals with HFpEF and HFrEF have been shown to have similar impairments in health-related quality of life, though evidence on sex differences is largely lacking.[25] In HFpEF participants enrolled in the Digitalis Investigation Group study, women had more symptoms and signs of HF compared with men. At time of enrollment, women were significantly more likely to have history of dyspnea at rest or orthopnea, edema, rales, or congestion on chest radiograph, and have worse New York Heart Association (NYHA) functional class.[26]

Hospitalization

Hospitalizations for HF are an important health consideration for the overall US population. In individuals age 55 years or older in the Atherosclerosis Risk in Communities (ARIC) cohort, the incidence rate of HF (ie, no prior history of HF) hospitalization was 11.6 per 1000 person-years. Furthermore, 55.3% of total cases occur in women, and 47.0% are for HFpEF.[1,27] In specifically evaluating HFpEF, 1.6 women per 1000 person-years had incident HFpEF in the WHI cohort.[6] Similarly, the estimated incidence of HFpEF was 2.4 women per 1000 person-years in a different set of cohorts.[5] Variation in incidence rate may be due to study populations, time periods, and outcome ascertainment.

Hospitalizations are an important outcome for individuals already diagnosed with HFpEF. In the Irbesartan in Heart Failure with Preserved Ejection Fraction (I-PRESERVE) cohort, women with HFpEF had an incidence rate of first all-cause hospitalization of 184.3 per 1000 person-years (**Table 1**).[28] Similarly, in the Candesartan in Heart failure: Assessment of Reduction in Mortality and morbidity (CHARM) cohort, the incidence rate for first all-cause hospitalization in women with HFpEF was 367.3 per 1000 person-years.[29] In these 2 cohorts, the incidence rate for men with HFpEF was 231.4 and 317.7 per 1000 person-years respectively, suggesting hospitalization rates were not significantly lower for women.[28,29] Moreover, recurrent hospitalizations occurred frequently. When participants were admitted with HFpEF, about 20% and 58% were readmitted in 30 days and 1 year.[30]

Women with HFpEF are hospitalized for a variety of causes. In the I-PRESERVE cohort, 54% of hospitalizations occurred for cardiovascular reasons, with the remainder being noncardiovascular causes. There are several risk factors for these hospitalizations. Women with increasing age (per year HR 1.024, 95% CI 1.014–1.035), obesity (HR 1.210, 95% CI 1.063–1.377), and DM (HR 1.454, 95% CI 1.128–1.872) were at relatively higher risk of mortality and/or hospitalization.[1,28] Notably,

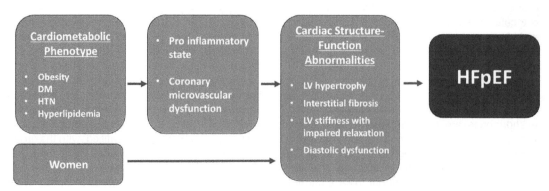

Fig. 2. Mechanistic pathways for HFpEF in women with cardiometabolic phenotype.

Table 1
Hospitalization and all-cause mortality rates (per 1000 person-years) for women and men with heart failure with preserved ejection fraction

	Women	Men
Hospitalizations (per 1000 person-y)	184–367	231–318
All-cause mortality (per 1000 person-y)	43–57	53–67

HFpEF is associated with significant morbidity and mortality. Rates of hospitalization and mortality are similar in women and men.

Variation in rates from different cohorts likely due to differences in study populations, time periods, and outcome ascertainment methods.

Data from Lam CS, Carson PE, Anand IS, et al. Sex differences in clinical characteristics and outcomes in elderly patients with heart failure and preserved ejection fraction: the Irbesartan in Heart Failure with Preserved Ejection Fraction (I-PRESERVE) trial. Circ Heart Fail 2012;5(5):571–8; and O'Meara E, Clayton T, McEntegart MB, et al. Sex differences in clinical characteristics and prognosis in a broad spectrum of patients with heart failure: results of the Candesartan in Heart failure: Assessment of Reduction in Mortality and morbidity (CHARM) program. Circulation 2007;115(24):3111–20.

these characteristics describe the cardiometabolic phenotype previously discussed. Additionally, noncardiovascular factors associated with mortality and hospitalization included COPD, anemia, and renal dysfunction.[28] Another study suggested AF was also associated with increased all-cause hospitalization (HR 1.63, 95% CI 1.40–1.91) and HF hospitalization (HR 1.54, 95% CI 1.15–2.06) in women with HFpEF.[31] Thus, women with HFpEF are often hospitalized, though further characterization of risk in specific phenotypes is needed.

Mortality

Mortality related to HF is of paramount concern. In 2015, HF was estimated to be the underlying cause in 75,251 deaths with 41,584 (55% of total) occurring in women. Any-mention, age-adjusted, death rate for HF in general population was 0.88 per 1000 person-years.[1] For HFpEF specifically, mortality rate has been evaluated in different study settings. A meta-analysis of 31 studies, including 10,347 participants with HFpEF, determined an all-cause mortality rate of 121 per 1000 person-years. When randomized controlled trials (RCTs) are excluded from the analysis to better represent a so-called real-world population, the mortality rate was 146 per 1000 person-years. Notably, in these analyses, the estimated mortality rate for HFrEF participants was significantly higher than for HFpEF participants.[32]

Certain studies report sex differences in mortality rates for HFpEF. In the I-PRESERVE cohort, all-cause mortality rate for women was 43.2 per 1000 person-years compared with 67.2 per 1000 person-years for men (relative risk 0.64, 95% CI 0.56–0.74).[28] However, in the CHARM cohort, all-cause mortality rate for women was 56.8 per 1000 person-years compared with 53.0 per 1000 person-years in men.[29] Therefore, even though mortality rates were comparable in these cohorts, sex differences in mortality need further investigation for more reliable results.

Most deaths in women with HFpEF occur due to cardiovascular causes. In the I-PRESERVE cohort, women with HFpEF had a cardiovascular mortality rate of 25.1 per 1000 person-years with 10.1 events per 1000 person-years due to sudden death. On the other hand, 12.6 deaths per 1000 person-years were due to noncardiovascular causes.[28] Similarly in the CHARM cohort, women with HFpEF had a cardiovascular mortality rate of 38.3 per 1000 person-years. HF and sudden death caused 11.9 and 12.5 deaths per 1000 person-years, respectively.[29]

There are several risk factors for mortality in women with HFpEF. As previously mentioned, the I-PRESERVE cohort established predictors of mortality and hospitalization in women. Therefore, the same risk factors of older age, obesity, DM, COPD, renal dysfunction, and anemia that identify the cardiometabolic phenotype potentially predispose women to increased risk of all-cause mortality.[28] AF is also a risk factor for cardiovascular mortality.[31] Likewise, an analysis of the GWTG cohort showed women with HFpEF at higher risk of in-hospital mortality have older age, COPD, renal dysfunction, and an increased heart rate.[33] Furthermore, recent hospitalization is an important risk factor for mortality. After an individual has been admitted for HFpEF, risk of mortality at 30 days and 1 year is 5% and 23%, respectively.[30] Overall, certain phenotypes and other risk factors, including prior hospitalization, are associated with increased risk of mortality in HFpEF in women, though causal mechanisms need to be further evaluated.

TREATMENT

Treatment of HFpEF remains challenging. Unlike HFrEF, which has several well established treatments supported by a robust evidence base and rigorous guidelines, HFpEF does not yet have a compelling evidence-based intervention proven to modify the natural history of this condition. The notable exception is spironolactone for which there are modest supportive data and a brief mention in the HF clinical practice guidelines.[4] Possible reasons for this discrepancy include trials with (1) improper patient selection, (2) inappropriately targeted therapies, and/or (3) inadequate treatments.[34] When considering treatment of HFpEF in women, evidence is even less given relatively smaller representation in trials and limited analysis of sex differences. Despite this, understanding of treatments in HFpEF has improved over the past several years.

Nonpharmacologic Treatments

As discussed, HFpEF is associated with comorbidities, including obesity, HTN, and renal dysfunction, that contribute to the pathogenesis. A management strategy for HFpEF includes treatment of these comorbidities, which may improve with nonpharmacologic measures such as dietary modifications and exercise training.

The role of caloric restriction and aerobic exercise training was studied in 100 obese, HFpEF participants, of which 80% are women and 95% have HTN. After 20 weeks, both interventions were associated with significant additive improvement in peak oxygen consumption and NYHA functional class.[35] Furthermore, the efficacy of a sodium-restricted dietary approaches to stop hypertension (DASH) diet in HFpEF participants with HTN and renal dysfunction has also been examined in a small cohort in which 13 out of 14 enrolled participants were women. After 21 days, participants had improved blood pressure, stroke volume, EF, and diastolic function.[36,37] Therefore, in these studies in which women were well-represented, dietary modifications and exercise training provided benefit in appropriately targeted HFpEF participants.

Pharmacologic Treatments

Pharmacotherapy is the cornerstone of guideline-directed medical therapy for HFrEF and includes diuretics, beta-blockers, renin-angiotensin-aldosterone system (RAAS) antagonists, and mineralocorticoid receptor antagonists (MRAs). The evidence is not as extensive for these medications in HFpEF. Recent evidence on sodium-glucose cotransporter 2 (SGLT2) inhibitors also suggests benefit for preventing HF in certain participants.

Volume overload is common in HFpEF, particularly in the cardiorenal phenotype.[34] Diuretics are instrumental in reducing intracardiac filling pressures, thereby having an American College of Cardiology (ACC)/AHA class I recommendation for symptomatic relief in HFpEF.[4,18] Diuretics can maintain renal perfusion and fluid homeostasis.

In addition to decongestion, the loop diuretic torsemide may affect myocardial collagen cross-linking, which would reduce fibrosis and improve LV diastolic function.[18]

Beta-blockers are a mainstay of HFrEF treatment, though evidence in HFpEF is less robust. A propensity-matched analysis of 8244 HFpEF participants from the Swedish Heart Failure Registry determined beta-blockers reduced all-cause mortality (HR 0.93, 95% CI 0.86–0.996) but showed no difference when mortality was combined with HF hospitalizations. Additionally, a subgroup analysis of 3774 women showed no significant difference between groups for all-cause mortality.[38] Thus, limited evidence does not provide justification for broadly using beta-blockers in women with HFpEF, though the medications may have utility in individuals with concomitant HTN, coronary heart disease, and/or AF.[4,18,34]

Angiotensin-converting enzyme (ACE) inhibitors and ARBs improve myocardial fibrosis, ventricular hypertrophy, and arterial stiffness. However, RCTs that evaluate these medications in HFpEF have not shown substantial benefit. These trials may have been underpowered and had high crossover rates.[34] The CHARM-Preserved trial randomized 3025 HFpEF participants, 40% women, to irbesartan or placebo. There was no significant difference in cardiovascular mortality but there was a reduction in HF hospitalizations (HR 0.84, 95% CI 0.70–1.00).[39] An analysis from the Swedish Heart Failure Registry demonstrated ACE inhibitors and ARBs in 6658 propensity-matched HFpEF participants was associated with reduced all-cause mortality (HR 0.91, 95% CI 0.85–0.98). However, a subgroup analysis in 3545 women showed no significant difference between groups.[40] The ACC/AHA guidelines discuss ACE inhibitors and ARBs in participants with HFpEF and HTN, and have a class IIb recommendation to consider ARBs for reduction in HFpEF hospitalizations.[4] Thus, there seems to be potential benefit of RAAS inhibition in certain HFpEF patients, though benefit in women is less evident.

Like RAAS inhibitors, MRAs reduce myocardial fibrosis and prevent myocardial remodeling. However, MRAs also affect collagen formation and extracellular matrix synthesis.[18,34] The Treatment of Preserved Cardiac Function Heart Failure with an Aldosterone Antagonist (TOPCAT) trial randomized participants to spironolactone or placebo. In a post hoc analysis of 1767 participants enrolled in the Americas, spironolactone was associated with reduced cardiovascular mortality (HR 0.74, 95% CI 0.57–0.97) and HF hospitalizations (HR 0.82, 95% CI 0.67–0.99).[41] Interestingly, a preliminary post hoc analysis showed spironolactone was associated with reduced all-cause mortality in 882 women in the Americas (HR 0.66, 95% CI 0.48–0.90), whereas a significant reduction was not seen in men.[42] The ACC/AHA guidelines have a class IIb recommendation to consider use of spironolactone in select HFpEF patients to reduce HF hospitalizations.[4] Overall, MRAs have shown potential benefit in treatment of HFpEF, though patient selection needs to be better defined.

Use of SGLT2 inhibitors may be useful in reducing cardiovascular outcomes in patients with DM. SGLT2 inhibitors induce glycosuria and natriuresis, thereby limiting volume overload. They may reduce myocardial hypertrophy, fibrosis, and remodeling.[43] Treatment with empagliflozin was associated with reduced HF hospitalization or cardiovascular death (HR 0.66, 95% CI 0.55–0.79), largely driven by a reduction in HF hospitalization (HR 0.65, 95% CI 0.50–85). In a subgroup analysis of 2004 women, differences remained significant. Notably, empagliflozin was not associated with a significant reduction in HF hospitalization in men.[44] Given biological plausibility and promising evidence thus far, SGLT2 inhibitors may have additional benefit for patients with HFpEF and DM, particularly in women. Multiple ongoing trials will provide more guidance on this issue.[43]

Neprilysin inhibition, via the drug sacubitril, has been a recent effective treatment of HFrEF and is being studied in HFpEF.[4,18] Neprilysin inhibition increases active natriuretic peptides and prevents breakdown of angiotensin. These effects have vasodilatory, natriuretic, and diuretic effects while also improving ventricular relaxation and reducing hypertrophy.[18,45] Sacubitril-valsartan was compared with valsartan in the phase 2 PARAMOUNT trial in 283 HFpEF participants, and demonstrated a significant reduction in N-terminal pro-BNP (not directly affected by neprilysin inhibition), which maintained significance in a subgroup analysis of women. The sacubitril-valsartan group also had improved NYHA functional class and decreased left atrial size.[45] Results from the large-scale Efficacy and Safety of LCZ696 Compared with Valsartan, on Morbidity and Mortality in Heart Failure Patients with Preserved Ejection Fraction (PARAGON-HF) should provide more definitive guidance.[18]

Personalized Medicine and Future Directions

HFpEF is a complex, multiorgan syndrome associated with adverse cardiovascular outcomes and limited treatment options.[8,34] HFpEF has multiple phenotypes (eg, cardiometabolic or cardiorenal)

based on patient characteristics, including sex.[23,24] Therapeutic strategies may need to be tailored to specific phenotypes, rather than a one-size-fits-all approach. For example, women with a cardiometabolic profile may benefit from an emphasis on caloric restriction, exercise training, MRAs, and/or SGLT2 inhibitors. Alternatively, the cardiorenal profile may be treated with sodium restriction, diuretics, and/or ultrafiltration. In addition, therapies can target comorbidities in HFpEF, such as revascularization for coronary heart disease or cardioversion for AF.[18,34–37,41,43] As phenotyping gets more sophisticated, it is evident that HFpEF has unique phenotypic profiles in women, which must be considered as treatments evolve.

Furthermore, certain mechanistic pathways can be targeted for treatments in HFpEF.[9,11,17] For example, statins are being investigated as a potential treatment for the proinflammatory state associated with certain phenotypes in HFpEF. Additionally, microvascular disease promotes reduction in nitric oxide and cyclic guanosine monophosphate, which in turn contributes to diastolic dysfunction and subsequent HFpEF. Inorganic nitrates or nitrites, soluble guanylate cyclase, and phosphodiesterase inhibitors are

---

Box 2
Ten unanswered questions about heart failure with preserved ejection fraction in women that can potentially be answered in future investigation

1. Why do men and women have similar incidence rates?

2. How does race affect risk of HFpEF in women?

3. What risk factors for HFpEF are different in women than men?

4. How can diagnosis of HFpEF in women be improved?

5. What is the role of sex hormones (eg, estrogen) in risk of HFpEF?

6. How can underlying mechanisms of HFpEF in women be better understood?

7. Can phenotypes of HFpEF in women be more precisely defined?

8. Can current therapies be effective in better defined patient populations?

9. Which future therapies will reduce hospitalizations and/or mortality?

10. How can novel therapeutic targets on mechanistic pathways be identified?

being evaluated as potential treatments targeting this pathway.[18,34] Although some of these pathways have been elucidated, a more thorough understanding is still needed. Overall, certain mechanisms are likely to predominate in particular phenotypes of HFpEF, and treatments should be developed, evaluated, and administered accordingly.[8,18,34]

SUMMARY

HFpEF is the most common form of HF in women and is associated with adverse clinical outcomes. Sex differences in the demographics, comorbidities, and underlying pathophysiology make phenotypes of HFpEF unique in women. Treatments thus far have not been overwhelmingly effective, though further investigation into more targeted therapies offers promise for the future (**Box 2**).

ACKNOWLEDGMENTS

The authors appreciate the helpful review by Sanjiv Shah, MD, Northwestern University, Feinberg School of Medicine.

REFERENCES

1. Benjamin EJ, Virani SS, Callaway CW, et al. Heart disease and stroke statistics-2018 update: a report from the American Heart Association. Circulation 2018;137(12):e67–492.
2. Steinberg BA, Zhao X, Heidenreich PA, et al. Trends in patients hospitalized with heart failure and preserved left ventricular ejection fraction: prevalence, therapies, and outcomes. Circulation 2012;126(1):65–75.
3. Owan TE, Redfield MM. Epidemiology of diastolic heart failure. Prog Cardiovasc Dis 2005;47(5):320–32.
4. Yancy CW, Jessup M, Bozkurt B, et al. 2017 ACC/AHA/HFSA focused update of the 2013 ACCF/AHA guideline for the management of heart failure: a report of the American College of Cardiology/American Heart Association Task Force on Clinical Practice Guidelines and the Heart Failure Society of America. Circulation 2017;136(6):e137–61.
5. Ho JE, Enserro D, Brouwers FP, et al. Predicting heart failure with preserved and reduced ejection fraction: the international collaboration on heart failure subtypes. Circ Heart Fail 2016;9(6) [pii: e003116].
6. Eaton CB, Pettinger M, Rossouw J, et al. Risk factors for incident hospitalized heart failure with preserved versus reduced ejection fraction in a multiracial cohort of postmenopausal women. Circ Heart Fail 2016;9(10) [pii:e002883].
7. Pandey A, Omar W, Ayers C, et al. Sex and race differences in lifetime risk of heart failure with preserved ejection fraction and heart failure with reduced ejection fraction. Circulation 2018;137(17):1814–23.
8. Borlaug BA. Heart failure with preserved and reduced ejection fraction: different risk profiles for different diseases. Eur Heart J 2013;34(19):1393–5.
9. Cheng S, Xanthakis V, Sullivan LM, et al. Correlates of echocardiographic indices of cardiac remodeling over the adult life course: longitudinal observations from the Framingham Heart Study. Circulation 2010;122(6):570–8.
10. Gori M, Lam CS, Gupta DK, et al. Sex-specific cardiovascular structure and function in heart failure with preserved ejection fraction. Eur J Heart Fail 2014;16(5):535–42.
11. Merz AA, Cheng S. Sex differences in cardiovascular ageing. Heart 2016;102(11):825–31.
12. Gupta DK, de Lemos JA, Ayers CR, et al. Racial differences in natriuretic peptide levels: the Dallas Heart Study. JACC Heart Fail 2015;3(7):513–9.
13. Chamberlain AM, St Sauver JL, Gerber Y, et al. Multimorbidity in heart failure: a community perspective. Am J Med 2015;128(1):38–45.
14. Saiki H, Petersen IA, Scott CG, et al. Risk of heart failure with preserved ejection fraction in older women after contemporary radiotherapy for breast cancer. Circulation 2017;135(15):1388–96.
15. Sharma K, Al Rifai M, Ahmed HM, et al. Usefulness of coronary artery calcium to predict heart failure with preserved ejection fraction in men versus women (from the Multi-Ethnic Study of Atherosclerosis). Am J Cardiol 2017;120(10):1847–53.
16. Lam CS, Lyass A, Kraigher-Krainer E, et al. Cardiac dysfunction and noncardiac dysfunction as precursors of heart failure with reduced and preserved ejection fraction in the community. Circulation 2011;124(1):24–30.
17. Paulus WJ, Tschope C. A novel paradigm for heart failure with preserved ejection fraction: comorbidities drive myocardial dysfunction and remodeling through coronary microvascular endothelial inflammation. J Am Coll Cardiol 2013;62(4):263–71.
18. Shah SJ, Kitzman DW, Borlaug BA, et al. Phenotype-specific treatment of heart failure with preserved ejection fraction: a multiorgan roadmap. Circulation 2016;134:73–90.
19. Hall PS, Nah G, Howard BV, et al. Reproductive factors and incidence of heart failure hospitalization in the women's health initiative. J Am Coll Cardiol 2017;69(20):2517–26.
20. Florijn BW, Bijkerk R, van der Veer EP, et al. Gender and cardiovascular disease: are sex-biased

microRNA networks a driving force behind heart failure with preserved ejection fraction in women? Cardiovasc Res 2018;114(2):210–25.

21. Zhao Z, Wang H, Jessup JA, et al. Role of estrogen in diastolic dysfunction. Am J Physiol Heart Circ Physiol 2014;306(5):H628–40.

22. Ebong IA, Watson KE, Goff DC Jr, et al. Age at menopause and incident heart failure: the Multi-Ethnic Study of Atherosclerosis. Menopause 2014; 21(6):585–91.

23. Shah SJ, Katz DH, Selvaraj S, et al. Phenomapping for novel classification of heart failure with preserved ejection fraction. Circulation 2015;131(3): 269–79.

24. Kao DP, Lewsey JD, Anand IS, et al. Characterization of subgroups of heart failure patients with preserved ejection fraction with possible implications for prognosis and treatment response. Eur J Heart Fail 2015;17(9):925–35.

25. Hoekstra T, Lesman-Leegte I, van Veldhuisen DJ, et al. Quality of life is impaired similarly in heart failure patients with preserved and reduced ejection fraction. Eur J Heart Fail 2011;13(9): 1013–8.

26. Deswal A, Bozkurt B. Comparison of morbidity in women versus men with heart failure and preserved ejection fraction. Am J Cardiol 2006;97(8): 1228–31.

27. Chang PP, Chambless LE, Shahar E, et al. Incidence and survival of hospitalized acute decompensated heart failure in four US communities (from the Atherosclerosis Risk in Communities Study). Am J Cardiol 2014;113(3):504–10.

28. Lam CS, Carson PE, Anand IS, et al. Sex differences in clinical characteristics and outcomes in elderly patients with heart failure and preserved ejection fraction: the Irbesartan in Heart Failure with Preserved Ejection Fraction (I-PRESERVE) trial. Circ Heart Fail 2012;5(5):571–8.

29. O'Meara E, Clayton T, McEntegart MB, et al. Sex differences in clinical characteristics and prognosis in a broad spectrum of patients with heart failure: results of the Candesartan in Heart failure: Assessment of Reduction in Mortality and morbidity (CHARM) program. Circulation 2007;115(24): 3111–20.

30. Nichols GA, Reynolds K, Kimes TM, et al. Comparison of risk of re-hospitalization, all-cause mortality, and medical care resource utilization in patients with heart failure and preserved versus reduced ejection fraction. Am J Cardiol 2015;116(7): 1088–92.

31. O'Neal WT, Sandesara P, Hammadah M, et al. Gender differences in the risk of adverse outcomes in patients with atrial fibrillation and heart failure with preserved ejection fraction. Am J Cardiol 2017; 119(11):1785–90.

32. Meta-analysis Global Group in Chronic Heart Failure (MAGGIC). The survival of patients with heart failure with preserved or reduced left ventricular ejection fraction: an individual patient data meta-analysis. Eur Heart J 2012;33(14): 1750–7.

33. Hsich EM, Grau-Sepulveda MV, Hernandez AF, et al. Sex differences in in-hospital mortality in acute decompensated heart failure with reduced and preserved ejection fraction. Am Heart J 2012;163(3): 430–7, 437.e1-3.

34. Senni M, Paulus WJ, Gavazzi A, et al. New strategies for heart failure with preserved ejection fraction: the importance of targeted therapies for heart failure phenotypes. Eur Heart J 2014; 35(40):2797–815.

35. Kitzman DW, Brubaker P, Morgan T, et al. Effect of caloric restriction or aerobic exercise training on peak oxygen consumption and quality of life in obese older patients with heart failure with preserved ejection fraction: a randomized clinical Trial. JAMA 2016;315(1):36–46.

36. Hummel SL, Seymour EM, Brook RD, et al. Low-sodium dietary approaches to stop hypertension diet reduces blood pressure, arterial stiffness, and oxidative stress in hypertensive heart failure with preserved ejection fraction. Hypertension 2012; 60(5):1200–6.

37. Hummel SL, Seymour EM, Brook RD, et al. Low-sodium DASH diet improves diastolic function and ventricular-arterial coupling in hypertensive heart failure with preserved ejection fraction. Circ Heart Fail 2013;6(6):1165–71.

38. Lund LH, Benson L, Dahlstrom U, et al. Association between use of beta-blockers and outcomes in patients with heart failure and preserved ejection fraction. JAMA 2014;312(19):2008–18.

39. Yusuf S, Pfeffer MA, Swedberg K, et al. Effects of candesartan in patients with chronic heart failure and preserved left-ventricular ejection fraction: the CHARM-Preserved Trial. Lancet 2003;362(9386): 777–81.

40. Lund LH, Benson L, Dahlstrom U, et al. Association between use of renin-angiotensin system antagonists and mortality in patients with heart failure and preserved ejection fraction. JAMA 2012;308(20): 2108–17.

41. Pfeffer MA, Claggett B, Assmann SF, et al. Regional variation in patients and outcomes in the Treatment of Preserved Cardiac Function Heart Failure With an Aldosterone Antagonist (TOPCAT) trial. Circulation 2015;131(1):34–42.

42. Kao DP, Flint KM, Merrill M. Spironolactone reduces all-cause mortality in women but not men with heart failure with preserved ejection fraction enrolled in TOPCAT from the Americas. Eur J Heart Fail 2017; 19(Suppl. S1):530.

43. Lytvyn Y, Bjornstad P, Udell JA, et al. Sodium glucose cotransporter-2 inhibition in heart failure: potential mechanisms, clinical applications, and summary of clinical trials. Circulation 2017;136(17):1643–58.

44. Fitchett D, Zinman B, Wanner C, et al. Heart failure outcomes with empagliflozin in patients with type 2 diabetes at high cardiovascular risk: results of the EMPA-REG OUTCOME(R) trial. Eur Heart J 2016; 37(19):1526–34.

45. Solomon SD, Zile M, Pieske B, et al. The angiotensin receptor neprilysin inhibitor LCZ696 in heart failure with preserved ejection fraction: a phase 2 double-blind randomised controlled trial. Lancet 2012; 380(9851):1387–95.

Heart Failure with Reduced Ejection Fraction in Women
Epidemiology, Outcomes, and Treatment

Gina Mentzer, MD[a],*, Eileen M. Hsich, MD[b]

KEYWORDS

- Systolic heart failure • Cardiomyopathies • Sex differences • Women

KEY POINTS

- Heart failure with reduced ejection fraction (HFrEF) affects more men than women but has significant morbidity and mortality for all patients.
- There are sex differences in the underlying disease causing HFrEF, with women more likely to have hypertension and valvular disease, and less likely to have coronary artery disease, than men.
- There are no sex-specific heart failure guidelines for medical management because women were underrepresented in clinical trials and the landmark trials were not prospectively designed to study sex differences.
- Post hoc and retrospective analysis suggest that β-blockers, aldosterone antagonists, angiotensin receptor blockers, and ivabradine are beneficial in all women with HFrEF, and the combination of hydralazine and isosorbide is beneficial in black women with HFrEF.
- Post hoc analysis suggests that sacubitril-valsartan is better than enalapril for women with HFrEF but it remains unclear if the benefit is due to valsartan or the combination of valsartan and sacubitril.

Heart failure is a constellation of symptoms and signs of fluid retention caused by abnormalities in the pericardium, myocardium, endocardium, heart valves, or coronary vessels. It is classified by the presence of an ejection fraction (EF) that is reduced (≤40%), borderline (41%–49%), or preserved (≥50%), and is associated with significant morbidity and mortality for both women and men.[1] It remains a leading cause of hospitalization and accounts for about 8% of all cardiovascular death.[2] There are many sex differences and this article focuses on those related to epidemiology, cause, diagnosis, medical therapy, and cardiac rehabilitation among heart failure patients with reduced EF.

EPIDEMIOLOGY, PROGNOSIS, AND CAUSES

Heart failure affects approximately 6.5 million adults in the United States, and nearly 50% of these are women. In 2013, approximately 500,000 new cases of heart failure occurred among women 55 years or older, with a similar but lower incidence among men.[2] Based on Olmsted County, Minnesota, data, the incidence of heart failure has declined over the years with a greater reduction in women with heart failure and reduced EF compared with men with heart failure and reduced or preserved EF (**Fig. 1**).[3] The prevalence of heart failure increases with age for both sexes with men more likely than women to have

Disclosure: The authors have nothing to disclose.
[a] Pioneer Heart Institute, Cardiovascular Clinic of Nebraska, LLC, Lincoln, NE 68526, USA; [b] Heart and Vascular Institute, Cleveland Clinic, Cleveland Clinic Lerner College of Medicine of Case Western Reserve University School of Medicine, 9500 Euclid Avenue, J3-4, Cleveland, OH 44195, USA
* Corresponding author.
E-mail address: gina.mentzer@gmail.com

Heart Failure Clin 15 (2019) 19–27
https://doi.org/10.1016/j.hfc.2018.08.003
1551-7136/19/© 2018 Elsevier Inc. All rights reserved.

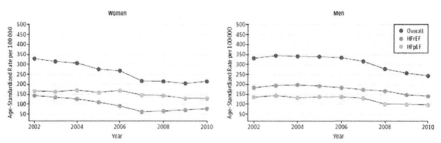

Fig. 1. Sex differences in incidence of heart failure with reduced EF (HFrEF) and heart failure with preserved EF (HFpEF). Data regarding the incidence of age-adjusted heart failure in Olmsted County, Minnesota, between January 1, 2000, and December 31, 2010, were stratified by sex and EF. The incidence of heart failure declined for both women and men but was greater in women with HFrEF compared with men with HFrEF or HFpEF. (*From* Gerber Y, Weston SA, Redfield MM, et al. A contemporary appraisal of the heart failure epidemic in Olmsted County, Minnesota, 2000 to 2010. JAMA Intern Med 2015;175(6):996–1004; with permission.)

heart failure with reduced EF (HFrEF). HFrEF is defined as an EF less than or equal to 40% and occurs in approximately 46% of those hospitalized with heart failure.[4] Compared with men, women hospitalized with HFrEF are more likely to be older, have hypertension and valvular disease, and less likely to have coronary artery disease or peripheral vascular disease.[5] There are no significant sex differences in in-hospital mortality among patients with HFrEF (2.69% women vs 2.89% men, $P = .20$) and women and men share many risk factors, including age, heart rate, systolic blood pressure, and history of renal failure or dialysis.[6] Approximately 40% of the patients hospitalized with HFrEF are women, and 5-year mortality for women and men with HFrEF is similar to heart failure patients with preserved EF (75.3% vs 75.7%, respectively).[4]

DIAGNOSIS

The diagnosis of HFrEF is defined by an EF less than or equal to 40% by imaging. According to the American College of Cardiology Foundation and American Heart Association heart failure guidelines, a 2-dimensional echocardiogram with Doppler should be performed on all heart failure patients to evaluate ventricular function, cardiac size, wall thickness and motion, and valve function during the initial evaluation and subsequent visits when there are changes in the clinical status or therapy expected to improve ventricular function. Cardiac MRI, cardiovascular computed tomography, nuclear stress testing, or cardiac catheterization may also be considered.[1] Based on population studies, including data from the Framingham Heart Study, HFrEF is less likely in women (**Fig. 2**).[7] In a recently published article by Shah and colleagues[4] involving more than 254 hospitals, women represented about 40% of patients hospitalized with HFrEF. The symptoms

and signs of heart failure are similar between women and men; however, women with HFrEF are more likely than men to have dyspnea, third heart sound (S3) gallop, jugular venous distension, and leg edema.[8]

BIOMARKERS

Biomarkers such as brain natriuretic peptide (BNP) or N-terminal pro-B-type natriuretic peptide (NT-proBNP) are useful to support clinical evaluation, diagnosis, and prognosis of heart failure, especially in cases in which uncertainty is present.[1] Women tend to have higher natriuretic peptide levels when compared with men with decompensated heart failure, including those with HFrEF (median BNP in women 1259 vs men 1113 pg/mL, $P<.001$). BNP is predictive of in-hospital mortality for both women and men almost regardless of the EF (**Table 1**).[5] The utility of serial

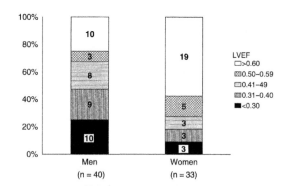

Fig. 2. Sex differences in left ventricular EF (LVEF) among subjects from the Framingham Heart Study who developed heart failure (*N* = 73). (*From* Vasan RS, Larson MG, Benjamin EJ, et al. Congestive heart failure in subjects with normal versus reduced left ventricular ejection fraction: prevalence and mortality in a population-based cohort. J Am Coll Cardiol 999;33(7):1948–50; with permission.)

Table 1
Sex differences in adjusted odds ratio for log brain natriuretic peptide and in-hospital mortality stratified by ejection fraction

| Odds Ratio | All Patients (N = 98,579) | EF <40% Female (n = 17,262) | Model 1, Adjusted Odds Ratio (95% CI), P Value | | | | |
			EF <40% Male (n = 29,171)	EF 40%–49% Female (n = 6666)	EF 40%–49% Male (n = 7085)	EF >50% Female (n = 24,907)	EF >50% Male (n = 13,488)
Unadjusted	1.45 (1.32–1.58), $P<.0001$	1.51 (1.23–1.86), $P = .0001$	1.48 (1.27–1.74), $P<.0001$	1.35 (1.04–1.75), $P = .0265$	1.28 (1.05–1.56), $P = .0163$	1.53 (1.38–1.71), $P<.0001$	1.32 (1.16–1.52), $P<.001$
Multivariate adjusted	1.34 (1.14–1.58), $P<.0004$	1.25 (0.97–1.61), $P = .0876$	1.28 (1.05–1.56), $P = .0161$	1.20 (0.84–1.71), $P = .3231$	1.18 (0.92–1.52), $P = .1857$	1.52 (1.34–1.71), $P<.0001$	1.25 (1.02–1.52), $P = .0291$

From Hsich EM, Grau-Sepulveda MV, Hernandez AF, et al. Relationship between sex, ejection fraction, and B-type natriuretic peptide levels in patients hospitalized with heart failure and associations with inhospital outcomes: findings from the get with the guideline-heart failure registry. Am Heart J 2013;166(6):1063–9; with permission.

measurements of natriuretic peptides can be helpful to guide optimal dosing of medical therapy with neurohormonal blocking agents, although sex-specific data are lacking.[1] An elevated troponin in the setting of chronic HFrEF portrays a poor prognosis for both women and men, especially when there is no significant coronary artery disease.[9] Newer biomarkers, such as soluble suppression of tumorigenicity 2 (ST2) and galactin-3, may have further potential for diagnosis, evaluation, and prognostic value; however, studies are still needed before routine clinical application.[10,11]

MEDICAL THERAPY

Over the last few decades, many HFrEF therapies have been proven to improve outcomes. Among the established medical therapies for HFrEF, angiotensin-converting enzyme inhibitors (ACEIs), angiotensin receptor blockers (ARBs), beta blockers, aldosterone antagonists, and hydralazine-isosorbide dinitrate have been shown in randomized controlled trials to improve symptoms, reduce burden of hospitalization, and decrease mortality.[1] Newer agents, such as angiotensin receptor-neprilysin inhibitor and the hyperpolarization channel blocker ivabradine, have recently been proven to be beneficial and added to the treatment guidelines for HFrEF.[12]

Currently, there are no HFrEF sex-specific guidelines because women have been underrepresented in clinical trials and sex-specific data were rarely prospectively analyzed. Female participation in landmark trials ranged from 0% to 40% with an average of about 20% women (**Table 2**).[13] One HFrEF trial to date, the Beta-Blocker Evaluation of Survival Trial (BEST),[14] has prospectively stratified patients by sex. All other studies either analyzed data retrospectively or via post hoc analysis.[13] This article summarizes the sex-specific data for all guideline HFrEF medical therapy based on the limited data available.

Table 2
Representation of women in heart failure with reduced ejection fraction clinical trials

Medical Therapy for HFrEF	Name	Trial (% Women, Number Women)
Beta blockers	Carvedilol	COPERNICUS[22] (20%, 469)
		US Carvedilol Study[21] (23%, 256)
	Metoprolol succinate	MERIT-HF[24] (23%, 898)
	Bisoprolol	CIBIS II[23] (19%, 515)
ACEI	Captopril, enalapril, ramipril, trandolapril, zofenopril	Meta-analysis[17] (19%, 2373)
	Captopril, enalapril, lisinopril, quinapril, ramipril	Meta-analysis[16] (23%, 1587)
ARB	Valsartan	Val-HeFT[19] (20%, 1003)
	Losartan	ELITE II[42] (31%, 966)
	Candesartan	CHARM—low EF[18] (26%, 1188)
Aldosterone antagonist or MRA	Eplerenone	EPHESUS[27] (29%, 1918)
		EMPHASIS-HF[26] (22%, 610)
	Spironolactone	RALES[25] (27%, 446)
Hydralazine or isosorbide dinitrate		V-HeFT I[28] (0%, 0)
		V-HeFT II[29] (0%, 0)
		A-HeFT[30] (40%, 420)
Digoxin		DIG[33] (22%, 1520)
Angiotensin receptor-neprilysin inhibitor	Sacubitril-valsartan	PARADIGM-HF[34] (22%, 1832)
Ivabradine		SHIFT[35] (23%, 1535)

Abbreviations: A-HeFT, African-American Heart Failure Trial; CHARM, Candesartan in Heart Failure Assessment of Mortality and Morbidity; CIBIS, Cardiac Insufficiency Bisoprolol Study; COPERNICUS, Carvedilol Prospective Randomized Cumulative Survival Study; DIG, Digitalis Investigation Group; ELITE, Evaluation of Losartan in the Elderly; ELITE EMPHASIS-HF, Eplerenone in Mild Patients Hospitalization and Survival Study in Heart Failure; EPHESUS, Eplerenone Post-Acute Myocardial Infarction Heart Failure Efficacy and Survival Study; MERIT-HF, Metoprolol Extended-Release Randomized Intervention Trial in Heart Failure; MRA, mineralocorticoid receptor antagonist; PARADIGM-HF, Prospective Comparison of ARNI with ACEI to Determine Impact on Global Mortality and Morbidity in Heart Failure; RALES, Randomized Aldactone Evaluation Study; SHIFT, Systolic Heart Failure Treatment with the I_f Inhibitor Ivabradine Trial; V-HeFT, Valsartan Heart Failure Trial.

Angiotensin-Converting Enzyme Inhibitors

ACEIs have been shown to be beneficial since the late 1980s when enalapril improved survival in patients with severe congestive heart failure when compared with placebo in the Cooperative North Scandinavian Enalapril Survival Study (CONSENSUS) trial.[15] ACEIs are recommended for all patients with HFrEF.[1] However, the benefits in women are unclear because too few women participated in the landmark trials. Two different large meta-analyses with more than 1500 women showed a trend toward improvement in survival and reduction in hospitalizations for women with HFrEF but no clear benefit because the 95% confidence intervals were wide and crossed 1.0.[16,17]

Angiotensin Receptor Blockers

ARBs are often used in ACEI-intolerant HFrEF patients, and deemed to have similar morbidity and mortality benefits.[12] Sex-specific data for ARBs are limited, with candesartan and valsartan appearing beneficial in women with HFrEF. Pooled data from 2 Candesartan in Heart Failure Assessment of Mortality and Morbidity (CHARM) trials (CHARM-Alternative to an ACEI and CHARM-Added to an ACEI) showed reduction of the combined endpoint of cardiovascular death or heart failure hospitalization for the 592 women with symptomatic heart failure and left ventricular EF less than or equal to 40% treated with candesartan when compared with the 596 women in the control group.[18] In the Valsartan Heart Failure Trial (Val-HeFT), valsartan was compared with placebo for patients with symptomatic HFrEF (EF ≤40%). Although valsartan did not significantly reduce mortality among women (N = 1003 women total in trial), it did reduce heart failure hospitalization with a hazard ratio (HR) of 0.74 (95% CI 0.55–0.98).[13,19]

Beta Blockers

Three beta-adrenergic receptor blockers (carvedilol, metoprolol succinate, and bisoprolol) are recommended and have been shown to improve survival in HFrEF with a relative risk reduction of mortality by about 30%.[1,20] Carvedilol is a nonselective, β-blocker with α-blocking and antioxidant properties. Trials such as the US Carvedilol Heart Failure Study and the Carvedilol Prospective Randomized Cumulative Survival Study (COPERNICUS) demonstrated benefit of carvedilol in women with symptomatic heart failure.[21,22] In the US Carvedilol Heart Failure Study, there were 256 women with HFrEF (EF ≤35%) and those treated with carvedilol had reduced mortality (HR 0.23, 95% CI 0.07–0.69).[21] In the COPERNICUS trial, which determined the effect of carvedilol in severely symptomatic patients with an EF less than 25%, carvedilol reduced the combined endpoint of death or hospitalization among the 469 women studied, mostly driven by a reduction in hospitalization.[22] Bisoprolol and metoprolol succinate are β-1 selective adrenergic antagonists that have proven benefit in HFrEF. The US Food and Drug Administration (FDA) approval was only for metoprolol succinate because bisoprolol was not studied in the United States. In the European Cardiac Insufficiency Bisoprolol Study (CIBIS II), bisoprolol improved all-cause mortality among the women participants (N = 515 women) when compared with controls.[23] In the Metoprolol Extended-Release Randomized Intervention Trial in Heart Failure (MERIT-HF), metoprolol succinate reduced heart failure hospitalization by 42% among women with symptomatic heart failure and an EF less than or equal to 40%, and by 72% in women with an EF less than 25%.[24]

Aldosterone Antagonists

Aldosterone antagonists are recommended for all HFrEF with symptoms and an EF less than or equal to 35% or an EF less than or equal to 40% after an acute myocardial infarction.[1] These drugs are quite favorable for women based on subgroup post hoc analysis as demonstrated by the Randomized Aldactone Evaluation Study (RALES), which included 446 women[25]; the Eplerenone in Mild Patients Hospitalization and Survival Study in Heart Failure (EMPHASIS-HF), which included 516 women[26]; and the Eplerenone Post-Acute Myocardial Infarction Heart Failure Efficacy and Survival Study (EPHESUS), which included 1918 women.[27] The RALES trial compared aldosterone to placebo in both ischemic and nonischemic heart failure patients with moderate-severe symptoms (New York Heart Association [NYHA] class III-IV) and an EF less than or equal to 35%, and demonstrated that women taking aldosterone had a reduction in mortality.[25] The EMPHASIS-HF study compared ischemic and nonischemic heart failure patients with mild symptoms (NYHA class II) and an EF less than 35% to eplerenone versus placebo. Among the women participants, the combined endpoint of mortality and heart failure hospitalization was reduced in those taking the drug.[26] The EPHESUS trial studied the effects of eplerenone among patients with an acute myocardial infarction and an EF less than or equal to 40%, and found women taking eplerenone had a reduction in mortality.[27]

Hydralazine-Isosorbide Dinitrate

The combination of hydralazine and isosorbide dinitrate in those who cannot tolerate an ACEI nor ARB was found to improve survival; however, this was only studied in men.[28,29] The only hydralazine and isosorbide dinitrate study that included women was the African-American Heart Failure Trial (A-HEFT), which was notable for enrolling 41% women (N = 420 women) with moderate-severe heart failure (NYHA class III-IV). This study demonstrated that the combination therapy improved survival, quality of life, and reduced hospitalization for African American women when added to ACEI or ARB and beta blockers.[30]

Digoxin

Since being first described in the 1700s to treat heart failure,[31] digoxin was commonly used and can be beneficial in reducing heart failure hospitalizations.[1] However, in the Digitalis Investigation Group (DIG) trial, the post hoc subgroup analysis demonstrated increased mortality in women with an adjusted HR of 1.23 (95% CI 1.02–1.47).[32] Most likely, this was due to increased serum levels of 1.2 to 2.0 ng/mL, with improved survival between 0.5 to 0.9 ng/mL for both sexes, in a retrospective analysis.[33] Given the lack of survival benefit with digoxin and the multiple benefits of other therapies, recommendations are to optimize other therapies before adding digoxin as current care.

Sacubitril-Valsartan

In 2014, the Prospective Comparison of ARNI [angiotensin receptor-neprilysin inhibitor] with ACEI to Determine Impact on Global Mortality and Morbidity in Heart Failure (PARADIGM-HF) trial results were published. It compared a neprilysin inhibitor (sacubitril) combined with an ARB (valsartan) versus an ACEI (enalapril) in symptomatic

heart failure patients (NYHA class II-IV) with an EF less than or equal to 40% (criteria amendment on Dec 15, 2010, changed to EF ≤35%). The PARADIGM-HF trial included 21% women (N = 1832) and demonstrated a reduction in the primary combined endpoint of cardiovascular mortality and heart failure hospitalization for women taking an ARNI when compared with women taking an ACEI. This benefit in women was driven by hospitalizations and not mortality (**Fig. 3**), raising the question of whether the neprilysin inhibitor added to the known benefit of valsartan to reduce hospitalization in women.[34] The ideal control for PARADIGM-HF would have been valsartan so that the effect of adding the neprilysin inhibitor could have been determined because the benefits of ACEI in women remain unclear.[17]

Ivabradine

Ivabradine was approved by the FDA in 2015 after the Systolic Heart Failure Treatment with the I_f Inhibitor Ivabradine Trial (SHIFT) trial in Europe demonstrated significant reduction in hospitalization for worsening heart failure. The trial included 23% women (N = 1535) in sinus rhythm who had chronic symptomatic systolic heart failure (NYHA class II-IV) with a resting heart rate greater than or equal to 70 beats per minute and an EF of less than or equal to 35%. A subgroup analysis on sex demonstrated similar effectiveness in women when compared with men.[35]

Antiplatelet Agents and Anticoagulation

The Studies of Left Ventricular Dysfunction (SOVLD) trial demonstrated that women had an increased risk of thromboembolic events compared with men, 2.4 events per 100 participant-years of follow-up versus 1.8 events per 100 participant-years of follow-up. The trial

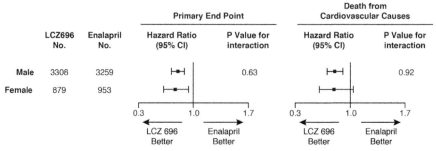

Fig. 3. Sex differences in outcome among HFrEF subjects in PARADIGM-HF taking sacubitril-valsartan (LCZ696) versus control therapy (enalapril). The combined primary endpoint was mortality and heart failure hospitalization. (*Adapted from* McMurray JJ, Packer M, Desai AS, et al. Angiotensin-neprilysin inhibition versus enalapril in heart failure. N Engl J Med 2014;371(11):993–1004; with permission.)

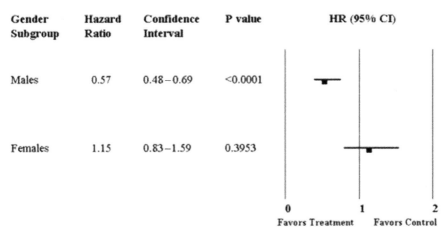

Gender Subgroup	Hazard Ratio	Confidence Interval	P value
Males	0.57	0.48–0.69	<0.0001
Females	1.15	0.83–1.59	0.3953

Fig. 4. Sex differences in HR for heart failure hospitalization among subjects with and without CardioMEMS. (*From* Loh JP, Barbash IM, Waksman R. Overview of the 2011 Food and Drug Administration Circulatory System Devices Panel of the Medical Devices Advisory Committee Meeting on the CardioMEMS Champion Heart Failure Monitoring System. J Am Coll Cardiol 2013;61(15):1571–5; with permission.)

was composed of 14% women (N = 921) with an EF less than or equal to 35%, and it excluded those with atrial fibrillation. A multivariable analysis noted sex differences in risk factors with a lower EF associated with higher risk of thromboembolic events in women but not in men. Usage of antiplatelet therapy was associated with a lower risk of thromboembolic events in both women and men although anticoagulant therapy was not. There were also sex differences in the type of thromboembolic events, with women having a higher percentage of pulmonary embolic events than men (24% vs 14%, P = .1).[36] To further explore prevention of thromboembolic events, the Warfarin versus Aspirin in Reduced Cardiac Ejection Fraction (WARCEF) trial was designed. The results showed no difference between agents in the risk of ischemic stroke, intracerebral hemorrhage, or death from any cause. The data were never analyzed for sex differences but did include 20% women (N = 461) with symptomatic HFrEF.[37]

Cardiac Rehabilitation

The Heart Failure: A Controlled Trial Investigating Outcomes of Exercise Training (HF-ACTION) trial included 28% women (N = 661) with symptomatic heart failure and an EF less than or equal to 35%. After adjustment for prognostic predictors, it demonstrated modest significant reductions in all-cause mortality or hospitalization, as well as in cardiovascular mortality or heart failure hospitalizations. Based on subgroup post hoc analysis, women benefited from an exercise training program and possibly more than men.[38]

CardioMEMS

The CardioMEMS (St Jude Medical-St Paul Tech Center, St. Paul, MN) is a device permanently implanted in the pulmonary artery to monitor pulmonary pressures to guide medical therapy for acute decompensated heart failure. The utility of the device was studied in the CardioMEMS Heart Sensor Allows Monitoring of Pressure to Improve Outcomes in NYHA Class III Patients (CHAMPION) study. CHAMPION was a single-blinded randomized controlled trial that included 78% (N = 431) HFrEF patients.[39] In a subgroup analysis of those with HFrEF that included 24% women (n = 111), treatment with the CardioMEMS demonstrated a 43% risk reduction in heart failure hospitalization and a 57% reduction in mortality.[40] The CHAMPION trial has been widely criticized for many reasons, including sex differences in outcomes. The FDA reviewed the analysis and did not consider the statistical methods adequate to account for the greater than expected variability in the primary endpoint of hospitalizations. Additionally, sex-specific data for the entire cohort (74% of total women were HFrEF), showed that the CardioMEMS reduced heart failure hospitalization in men but not women (**Fig. 4**), although the sponsors stated that the study was inadequately powered to detect sex differences due to the small number of events in women.[41]

SUMMARY

HFrEF is less common in women than men but with several sex differences in the underlying disease. Women with HFrEF are more likely than men to have hypertension and valvular disease, and less likely to have coronary artery disease.

In-hospital mortality is similar and low; however, when hospitalized for acute decompensated heart failure, the 5-year mortality rate is very high for both men and women. Natriuretic peptide serum levels are higher in women with decompensated heart failure than men but yield similar prognostic risk for in-hospital mortality. The CardioMEMS is used to monitor acute decompensated heart failure events and guide therapy, although their utility in women remains unclear based on information from the CHAMPION trial. There remains no sex-specific guideline therapy for HFrEF because women were underrepresented in clinical trials and studies were never designed to prospectively study sex differences. Based on post hoc analyses or retrospective studies, β-blockers, aldosterone antagonists, ARBs, and ivabradine seem beneficial in women with HFrEF. The combination of hydralazine and isosorbide was studied in black women with HFrEF and found to reduce mortality, reduce hospitalizations, and improve quality of life. More studies are needed and should be prospectively designed to study sex differences to better understand the effects of drugs and technology on women with HFrEF.

ACKNOWLEDGMENTS

Eileen Hsich is supported by the National Heart, Lung and Blood Institute of the National Institute of Health under Award Number R01HL141892. The content is solely the responsibility of the authors and does not necessarily represent the official views of the National Institutes of Health.

REFERENCES

1. Yancy CW, Jessup M, Bozkurt B, et al. 2013 ACCF/AHA guideline for the management of heart failure: a report of the American College of Cardiology Foundation/American Heart Association Task Force on practice guidelines. Circulation 2013;128(16): e240–327.
2. Benjamin EJ, Blaha MJ, Chiuve SE, et al. Heart disease and stroke statistics-2017 update: a report from the American Heart Association. Circulation 2017;135(10):e146–603.
3. Gerber Y, Weston SA, Redfield MM, et al. A contemporary appraisal of the heart failure epidemic in Olmsted County, Minnesota, 2000 to 2010. JAMA Intern Med 2015;175(6):996–1004.
4. Shah KS, Xu H, Matsouaka RA, et al. Heart failure with preserved, borderline, and reduced ejection fraction: 5-year outcomes. J Am Coll Cardiol 2017; 70(20):2476–86.
5. Hsich EM, Grau-Sepulveda MV, Hernandez AF, et al. Relationship between sex, ejection fraction, and B-type natriuretic peptide levels in patients hospitalized with heart failure and associations with inhospital outcomes: findings from the Get With The Guideline-Heart Failure Registry. Am Heart J 2013; 166(6):1063–71.e3.
6. Hsich EM, Grau-Sepulveda MV, Hernandez AF, et al. Sex differences in in-hospital mortality in acute decompensated heart failure with reduced and preserved ejection fraction. Am Heart J 2012;163(3): 430–7, 437.e1-3.
7. Vasan RS, Larson MG, Benjamin EJ, et al. Congestive heart failure in subjects with normal versus reduced left ventricular ejection fraction: prevalence and mortality in a population-based cohort. J Am Coll Cardiol 1999;33(7):1948–55.
8. Johnstone D, Limacher M, Rousseau M, et al. Clinical characteristics of patients in Studies of Left Ventricular Dysfunction (SOLVD). Am J Cardiol 1992; 70(9):894–900.
9. Egstrup M, Schou M, Tuxen CD, et al. Prediction of outcome by highly sensitive troponin T in outpatients with chronic systolic left ventricular heart failure. Am J Cardiol 2012;110(4):552–7.
10. Chow SL, Maisel AS, Anand I, et al. Role of biomarkers for the prevention, assessment, and management of heart failure: a scientific statement from the American Heart Association. Circulation 2017;135(22):e1054–91.
11. Motiwala SR, Sarma A, Januzzi JL, et al. Biomarkers in ACS and heart failure: should men and women be interpreted differently? Clin Chem 2014;60(1):35–43.
12. Yancy CW, Jessup M, Bozkurt B, et al. 2016 ACC/AHA/HFSA focused update on new pharmacological therapy for heart failure: an update of the 2013 ACCF/AHA Guideline for the Management of Heart Failure: a report of the American College of Cardiology/American Heart Association Task Force on Clinical Practice Guidelines and the Heart Failure Society of America. Circulation 2016;134(13):e282–93.
13. Hsich EM, Pina IL. Heart failure in women: a need for prospective data. J Am Coll Cardiol 2009;54(6):491–8.
14. Ghali JK, Krause-Steinrauf HJ, Adams KF, et al. Gender differences in advanced heart failure: insights from the BEST study. J Am Coll Cardiol 2003;42(12):2128–34.
15. CONSENSUS Trial Study Group. Effects of enalapril on mortality in severe congestive heart failure. Results of the Cooperative North Scandinavian Enalapril Survival Study (CONSENSUS). N Engl J Med 1987;316(23):1429–35.
16. Garg R, Yusuf S. Overview of randomized trials of angiotensin-converting enzyme inhibitors on mortality and morbidity in patients with heart failure. Collaborative Group on ACE Inhibitor Trials. JAMA 1995;273(18):1450–6.
17. Shekelle PG, Rich MW, Morton SC, et al. Efficacy of angiotensin-converting enzyme inhibitors and

beta-blockers in the management of left ventricular systolic dysfunction according to race, gender, and diabetic status: a meta-analysis of major clinical trials. J Am Coll Cardiol 2003;41(9):1529–38.

18. Young JB, Dunlap ME, Pfeffer MA, et al. Mortality and morbidity reduction with Candesartan in patients with chronic heart failure and left ventricular systolic dysfunction: results of the CHARM low-left ventricular ejection fraction trials. Circulation 2004; 110(17):2618–26.

19. Cohn JN, Tognoni G. A randomized trial of the angiotensin-receptor blocker valsartan in chronic heart failure. N Engl J Med 2001;345(23):1667–75.

20. Fonarow GC, Yancy CW, Hernandez AF, et al. Potential impact of optimal implementation of evidence-based heart failure therapies on mortality. Am Heart J 2011;161(6):1024–30.e3.

21. Packer M, Bristow MR, Cohn JN, et al. The effect of carvedilol on morbidity and mortality in patients with chronic heart failure. U.S. Carvedilol Heart Failure Study Group. N Engl J Med 1996;334(21):1349–55.

22. Packer M, Fowler MB, Roecker EB, et al. Effect of carvedilol on the morbidity of patients with severe chronic heart failure: results of the carvedilol prospective randomized cumulative survival (COPERNICUS) study. Circulation 2002;106(17):2194–9.

23. Simon T, Mary-Krause M, Funck-Brentano C, et al. Sex differences in the prognosis of congestive heart failure: results from the Cardiac Insufficiency Bisoprolol Study (CIBIS II). Circulation 2001;103(3): 375–80.

24. Ghali JK, Pina IL, Gottlieb SS, et al. Metoprolol CR/XL in female patients with heart failure: analysis of the experience in Metoprolol Extended-Release Randomized Intervention Trial in Heart Failure (MERIT-HF). Circulation 2002;105(13):1585–91.

25. Pitt B, Zannad F, Remme WJ, et al. The effect of spironolactone on morbidity and mortality in patients with severe heart failure. Randomized Aldactone Evaluation Study Investigators. N Engl J Med 1999;341(10):709–17.

26. Zannad F, McMurray JJ, Krum H, et al. Eplerenone in patients with systolic heart failure and mild symptoms. N Engl J Med 2011;364(1):11–21.

27. Pitt B, Remme W, Zannad F, et al. Eplerenone, a selective aldosterone blocker, in patients with left ventricular dysfunction after myocardial infarction. N Engl J Med 2003;348(14):1309–21.

28. Cohn JN, Archibald DG, Ziesche S, et al. Effect of vasodilator therapy on mortality in chronic congestive heart failure. Results of a Veterans Administration Cooperative Study. N Engl J Med 1986; 314(24):1547–52.

29. Cohn JN, Johnson G, Ziesche S, et al. A comparison of enalapril with hydralazine-isosorbide dinitrate in the treatment of chronic congestive heart failure. N Engl J Med 1991;325(5):303–10.

30. Taylor AL, Lindenfeld J, Ziesche S, et al. Outcomes by gender in the African-American Heart Failure Trial. J Am Coll Cardiol 2006;48(11):2263–7.

31. Dodsley J, Elmsly P, Leigh Sotheby. Medical transactions, Vol. 3. College of Physicians in London; 1785.

32. Rathore SS, Wang Y, Krumholz HM. Sex-based differences in the effect of digoxin for the treatment of heart failure. N Engl J Med 2002;347(18): 1403–11.

33. Adams KF Jr, Patterson JH, Gattis WA, et al. Relationship of serum digoxin concentration to mortality and morbidity in women in the digitalis investigation group trial: a retrospective analysis. J Am Coll Cardiol 2005;46(3):497–504.

34. McMurray JJ, Packer M, Desai AS, et al. Angiotensin-neprilysin inhibition versus enalapril in heart failure. N Engl J Med 2014;371(11):993–1004.

35. Swedberg K, Komajda M, Bohm M, et al. Ivabradine and outcomes in chronic heart failure (SHIFT): a randomised placebo-controlled study. Lancet 2010;376(9744):875–85.

36. Dries DL, Rosenberg YD, Waclawiw MA, et al. Ejection fraction and risk of thromboembolic events in patients with systolic dysfunction and sinus rhythm: evidence for gender differences in the Studies of Left Ventricular dysfunction trials. J Am Coll Cardiol 1997;29(5):1074–80.

37. Homma S, Thompson JL, Pullicino PM, et al. Warfarin and aspirin in patients with heart failure and sinus rhythm. N Engl J Med 2012;366(20): 1859–69.

38. O'Connor CM, Whellan DJ, Lee KL, et al. Efficacy and safety of exercise training in patients with chronic heart failure: HF-ACTION randomized controlled trial. JAMA 2009;301(14):1439–50.

39. Abraham WT, Adamson PB, Bourge RC, et al. Wireless pulmonary artery haemodynamic monitoring in chronic heart failure: a randomised controlled trial. Lancet 2011;377(9766):658–66.

40. Givertz MM, Stevenson LW, Costanzo MR, et al. Pulmonary artery pressure-guided management of patients with heart failure and reduced ejection fraction. J Am Coll Cardiol 2017;70(15): 1875–86.

41. Loh JP, Barbash IM, Waksman R. Overview of the 2011 Food and drug administration circulatory system devices panel of the medical devices advisory committee meeting on the CardioMEMS champion heart failure monitoring system. J Am Coll Cardiol 2013;61(15):1571–6.

42. Pitt B, Poole-Wilson PA, Segal R, et al. Effect of losartan compared with captopril on mortality in patients with symptomatic heart failure: randomised trial—the Losartan Heart Failure Survival Study ELITE II. Lancet 2000;355(9215):1582–7.

Peripartum Cardiomyopathy
Progress in Understanding the Etiology, Management, and Prognosis

Kathryn J. Lindley, MD[a,*], Amanda K. Verma, MD[a],
Lori A. Blauwet, MD[b]

KEYWORDS

- Peripartum cardiomyopathy • Heart failure • Pregnancy • Diagnosis • Prognosis

KEY POINTS

- PPCM is an idiopathic cardiomyopathy occurring in women near the end of pregnancy or within 5 months after delivery.
- Preeclampsia, black race, multiparity, and multiple gestation are risk factors.
- PPCM is likely caused by a complex interaction of genetic and environmental factors.
- Up to 72% of women with PPCM have improvement in LVEF, but increased LV remodeling, black race, and initial LVEF less than 30% are poor prognostic factors.
- Subsequent pregnancy is associated with significant risk of recurrent heart failure and mortality in women with persistent LV dysfunction.

HISTORY AND DEFINITION

First described in the literature in the 1800s, peripartum cardiomyopathy (PPCM) was observed but not well understood for decades (**Table 1**).[1–4] The term "peripartum cardiomyopathy" was first coined and diagnostic criteria first published in 1971.[5] The diagnostic criteria were further refined by a National Heart, Lung, and Blood Institute and Office of Rare Diseases (National Institutes of Health) workshop in 2000[6] and modified by the Heart Failure Association of the European Society of Cardiology Working Group on Peripartum Cardiomyopathy in 2010.[7]

Epidemiology

Given the variation in diagnostic criteria and likelihood of underdiagnosis because of lack of awareness of this disease, the true incidence of PPCM remains unknown. Incidence has been reported as 1 in 300 live births in Haitian women and 1 in 20,000 live births in Japan.[8,9] The Nationwide Inpatient Sample database has identified an incidence of approximately 1 in 1000 live births in the United States.[10] African American women have the highest incidence and Hispanic women the lowest.[10,11] A recent study reported that African Americans were diagnosed at a younger age and later in the postpartum period, and showed more significant left ventricular (LV) dysfunction at diagnosis than non–African American women.[12]

Presentation

Women typically present with heart failure (HF) symptoms in the last gestational month or within 5 months after delivery, although patients may

Disclosure: The authors have nothing to disclose.
[a] Cardiovascular Division, Washington University in St. Louis, 660 South Euclid Avenue, Box 8086, St Louis, MO 63110, USA; [b] Cardiovascular Medicine, Mayo Clinic, 200 1st Street Southwest, Rochester, MN 55905, USA
* Corresponding author.
E-mail address: kathryn.lindley@wustl.edu

heartfailure.theclinics.com

Table 1
History of PPCM

Author(s), Year	Author Location/ Affiliation	Significance	Quote
Meigs,[1] 1848	Jefferson Medical College at Philadelphia, Philadelphia, Pennsylvania	First published description of PPCM	She presented all the appearances of great dilation of the auricles and ventricles of the heart....the respiration was troubled...the lower limbs became considerably infiltrated....[she] could not lie down day or night...it was difficult to imagine that the heart could ever recover...after the birth of her child, her health soon became stronger, and now she is in consummate health. The heart presents no evidences of disease whatever.
Hull & Hafkesbring,[2] 1937	Louisiana State University Medical Center, New Orleans, Louisiana	First published PPCM case series (27 patients)	...there is a type of heart disease which is correlated with events that transpired during pregnancy or shortly after its termination. To this type the name "toxic" postpartal heart disease has tentatively been given. "Toxic" postpartal heart disease presents a fairly characteristic clinical picture, and seems to constitute a fairly definite clinical entity.
Gouley et al,[3] 1937	Perelman School of Medicine, University of Pennsylvania, Philadelphia, Pennsylvania	Autopsy series of 4 PPCM cases	...necropsy showed a myocardial degeneration differing from the lesions ordinarily associated with the current classification of heart disease. The coronary arteries were normal...Death occurred in three cases following embolism, which had its origin on the endocardial surface of degenerated heart muscle.
Meadows,[4] 1957	Cook County Hospital, Chicago, Illinois	Stressed importance of ruling out other heart failure etiologies, such as hypertension and rheumatic heart disease	The purpose of this report is to confirm and extend previous observations made on this syndrome and to stress the absence of previous heart disease or hypertension in most of these cases. These instances also add further basis for the belief of previous observers that the coincidental pregnancy is in some way related to the myocardiopathy and suggest that many of these cases may be misdiagnosed as rheumatic or hypertensive heart disease due to the lack of general recognition of the syndrome.

(continued on next page)

	Author Location/		
Author(s), Year	Affiliation	Significance	Quote
Demakis & Rahimtoola,[5] 1971	Cook County Hospital, Chicago, Illinois, and University of Illinois College of Medicine, Chicago, Illinois	First published diagnostic criteria for PPCM	The criteria for the diagnosis of PPCM are (1) development of heart failure in the last month of pregnancy or within the first 5 postpartum months, (2) absence of a determinable etiology for the cardiac failure, and (3) absence of demonstrable heart disease prior to the last month of pregnancy.
Pearson et al,[6] 2000	National Heart, Lung, and Blood Institute and the Office of Rare Diseases of the National Institutes of Health	Expanded PPCM diagnostic criteria to include specific echo criteria defining LV systolic dysfunction	• Development of cardiac failure in the last month of pregnancy or within 5 mo of delivery • Absence of an identifiable cause for the cardiac failure • Absence of recognizable heart disease before the last month of pregnancy • LV systolic dysfunction demonstrated by classical echocardiographic criteria: ejection fraction <45% or fractional shortening <30%, or both
Sliwa et al,[7] 2010	Heart Failure Association of the European Society of Cardiology Working Group on Peripartum Cardiomyopathy	Revised criteria for timing of presentation, added statement regarding LV chamber size and modified LV systolic dysfunction criteria	PPCM is an idiopathic cardiomyopathy presenting with heart failure secondary to LV systolic dysfunction toward the end of pregnancy or in the months following delivery, where no other cause of heart failure is found. It is a diagnosis of exclusion. The left ventricle may not be dilated but the ejection fraction is nearly always reduced below 45%.

Abbreviation: LV, left ventricular.

present at earlier gestational ages.[12,13] Most women are diagnosed the first week after delivery.[12,13] Reports suggest that presentation before delivery may be associated with worse prognosis, including lower rate of LV ejection fraction (LVEF) recovery.[14] Preeclampsia has been identified as a risk factor for PPCM, with the prevalence of preeclampsia among women with PPCM more than four times the worldwide background rate.[15] Multigravity/multiparity, multiple gestation, African descent, and low socioeconomic status have also been associated with increased risk for PPCM.[15,16]

A high index of suspicion is necessary for the expedient diagnosis of PPCM, because many symptoms of HF mimic symptoms commonly occurring during normal pregnancy.[7,17] Delay of diagnosis for more than 1 week from the onset of

symptoms is common and is associated with increased risk of major adverse events.[17] Thus, awareness of PPCM is important and prompt evaluation should be pursued if HF symptoms occur.[17]

Patients with PPCM often present with New York Heart Association (NYHA) functional class III-IV symptoms, including progressive dyspnea, reduced exercise tolerance, lower extremity edema, paroxysmal nocturnal dyspnea, orthopnea, and cough.[7] On examination, elevated jugular venous pressure, an S3 heart sound, a holosystolic mitral regurgitation murmur, rales, and peripheral edema may be observed.[18,19]

Diagnosis

B-type natriuretic peptide (BNP) may be a helpful screening test for PPCM. Although BNP levels are normal in uncomplicated pregnancy, BNP or N-terminal-proBNP levels are elevated in women with PPCM, and N-terminal-proBNP levels correlate with clinical outcomes, including recovery of LVEF.[7,20]

Echocardiographic identification of LVEF less than 45% is necessary for the diagnosis of PPCM.[6,7] In the Investigations of Pregnancy-Associated Cardiomyopathy (IPAC) study, the mean LVEF at study entry was 35%, and was significantly lower in black compared with nonblack women.[11] The LV is often, but not always, dilated.[7] Different patterns of LV remodeling have been reported in PPCM associated with preeclampsia, with smaller LV end-diastolic diameter and less eccentric remodeling than in women without preeclampsia.[21]

No specific cardiovascular magnetic resonance pattern has been identified in women with PPCM, but right ventricular (RV) dysfunction, focal nonischemic late gadolinium enhancement, and regional wall motion abnormalities have been described.[22,23] Increased LV T2 ratio and early gadolinium enhancement ratio have been reported during the acute stage of PPCM, consistent with myocardial inflammation.[24,25] Small studies suggest that late gadolinium enhancement may be associated with worse prognosis.[24–26]

POSSIBLE ETIOLOGIES AND PATHOPHYSIOLOGY
Genetics and Dilated Cardiomyopathy

Familial clustering of PPCM is described in case reports.[27,28] Increased incidence of idiopathic dilated cardiomyopathy (IDCM) is also reported in families with PPCM, suggesting that IDCM and PPCM may represent different points along a spectrum of cardiomyopathic disease.[29,30] Several genetic studies suggest that truncating variants in the gene encoding the protein titin may be responsible for predisposition for development of either PPCM or IDCM.[30,31] A recent study of PPCM patients identified 26 truncating variants in eight genes that have previously been associated with IDCM, most involving the gene encoding titin.[30] These truncating variants affected PPCM patients in a higher proportion (15%) than in the general population (4.7%).[30] A polymorphism of guanine nucleotide-binding proteins β-3 that leads to the "TT genotype" is more prevalent in black persons compared with nonblack persons with PPCM and is associated with lower likelihood of recovery.[32]

Immune-Mediated Mechanisms

The immune system is shifted to enhance humoral immunity and to suppress adaptive immunity to maintain pregnancy. In PPCM, this shift in immunity may be altered such that adaptive immunity is favored, which may lead to cardiac dysfunction. Compared with pregnancy-matched healthy control subjects, patients with PPCM have reduced expression of costimulatory receptor PD-1 and its ligand B7-H1, which normally facilitate enhancement of humoral immunity during pregnancy.[33–35] Patients with PPCM also have abnormal expression of downstream cytokines, including an elevated level of interferon-γ (a result of adaptive immunity) and decreased level of interleukin-4 (a result of humoral immunity).[35] Patients enrolled in the IPAC study had decreased levels of natural killer cells and increased levels of T-double negative cells expressing CD38.[36] Because natural killer cells are responsible for destruction of virus-infected cells, a viral-mediated process may possibly provoke PPCM. The role of T-double negative cells in PPCM remains unclear at this time.

Microchimerism is observed during pregnancy and may play a role in the development of PPCM via an autoimmune reaction. Fetal microchimeric stem cells can hypothetically differentiate into dendritic cells, which process maternal cardiac antigens and provoke an autoimmune response. In a small study of women with PPCM who had delivered males, there were higher levels of male DNA in the mother's blood compared with the blood of non-PPCM control subjects.[37] Detectable levels of antibodies to cardiac antigens were identified in sera of PPCM patients that were not found in sera of control subjects, including healthy women after pregnancy, nonpregnant women, and IDCM.[37]

If an immune-mediated pathway is a pathophysiologic mechanism of PPCM, a stimulus would be required to trigger such response. Historically, this stimulus was thought to be a virus. In a study of 26 women with PPCM, virus detection was no different than in control subjects, but histology of endomyocardial biopsies from patients with PPCM exclusively had inflammatory findings.[38]

Angiogenic Imbalance

There is growing interest in angiogenic imbalance as a possible cause of PPCM.[39–41] During normal pregnancy, a dynamic angiogenic environment allows for placental development and embryogenesis to occur, with a shift toward antiangiogenesis in late pregnancy. In PPCM, there is an exaggerated shift toward antiangiogenesis, potentially contributing to endothelial dysfunction and microvascular ischemia. The "two hit" hypothesis describes how excessive antiangiogenic signals occurring late in pregnancy, coupled with the host's inability to tolerate a vasculotoxic environment, leads to increased risk for PPCM.[39–41] Signal transducer and activator of transcription 3 is a transcription factor that reduces oxidative stress by regulation of mitochondrial superoxide dismutase (MNSOD). Peroxisome proliferator-activated receptor gamma coactivator 1-α is a transcription factor that drives mitochondrial biogenesis and induces expression of proangiogenic factors, including vascular endothelial growth factor (VEGF). In murine models, absence of signal transducer and activator of transcription 3 and underexpression of peroxisome proliferator-activated receptor gamma coactivator 1-α were independently associated with suppression of MNSOD and an increase in reactive oxygen species.[39,42] Suppression of MNSOD leads to inappropriate cleavage of prolactin by cathepsin D into an antiangiogenic 16-kDa fragment that causes vascular endothelial and cardiomyocyte dysfunction and apoptosis.[42]

The placenta secretes high levels of antiangiogenic factors in the third trimester, including soluble fms-like tyrosine kinase 1 (sFLT1).[39] sFLT1 is a soluble VEGF receptor that binds to proangiogenic VEGF and placental growth factor, preventing these factors from binding to cell-surface receptors, ultimately causing endothelial dysfunction.[39] sFLT1, 16-kDa prolactin, placental growth factor, and VEGF levels have been shown to differ in women with PPCM compared with healthy control subjects in animal and human studies.[39,43,44] Higher sFLT1 levels in women with PPCM have been associated with worse NYHA functional class and decreased survival.[44]

Recent investigations have strengthened the association of preeclampsia with PPCM.[15] Although sFLT1 levels rise during the third trimester of all pregnancies, levels are markedly elevated during preeclamptic pregnancies.[45–47] Preeclampsia and PPCM may thus share common pathogenic pathways via angiogenic imbalance.[15] Further investigation into this potential relationship is warranted.

TREATMENT/MANAGEMENT
Heart Failure Medications

Given the paucity of clinical trials, current guidelines on the management of PPCM are based on expert consensus opinion.[48] Initial management should be multidisciplinary, considering the health of mother and fetus.[7] Guideline-directed medical therapy (GDMT) for HF with reduced LVEF, adjusted for concerns regarding risk of fetal

toxicity in the antepartum period and transmission of drug to baby when breastfeeding, should be initiated as soon as possible.

Antepartum, angiotensin-converting enzyme inhibitors and angiotensin receptor blockers should be avoided.[49] Instead, hydralazine and nitrates may be prescribed for afterload reduction.[49] Postpartum, patients are transitioned to an angiotensin-converting enzyme inhibitor or angiotensin receptor blockers. Enalapril or captopril are preferred if the patient is breastfeeding.[50] β-Blockers are safe during pregnancy and while breastfeeding. Mineralocorticoids should only be used postpartum.[49] Diuretics should be used cautiously in the antepartum patient to reduce the risk of placental hypoperfusion with overdiuresis.[7] There are limited data suggesting benefit from ivabradine or sacubitril/valsartan in patients with PPCM.[51–53] Sacubitril/valsartan is contraindicated during pregnancy.[54] There are limited data regarding the safety of ivabradine during pregnancy and the safety of sacubitril/valsartan and ivabradine while breastfeeding.[50,55]

Bromocriptine

Bromocriptine has been proposed as a novel treatment of PPCM. Bromocriptine inhibits the release of prolactin, thus preventing the creation of the cleaved 16-kDa fragment implicated in the pathogenesis of PPCM. In a prospective, randomized, open-label, proof-of-concept pilot study, women with PPCM and LVEF less than or equal to 35% received GDMT for HF or GDMT for HF plus bromocriptine for 8 weeks.[56] Patients who received bromocriptine had significantly greater recovery of LVEF, greater improvement in NYHA functional class, and decreased mortality at 6-month follow-up compared with those who received GDMT alone.[56] These results were not confirmed in a German PPCM cohort, of whom 67% were treated with bromocriptine. The percentage of patients experiencing full recovery was similar in both groups, with no difference in baseline characteristics.[57]

A recent multicenter study of 63 PPCM patients with LVEF less than or equal to 35% at diagnosis compared outcomes among women randomized to either 1 week or 8 weeks of treatment with bromocriptine. There was no significant difference in recovery of LVEF or HF hospitalizations based on treatment duration.[58] Because the incremental benefit of bromocriptine in addition to GDMT has yet to be determined, there are currently no specific recommendations regarding use of this medication in PPCM patients.

Anticoagulation

Anticoagulation should be strongly considered in PPCM patients if LVEF is less than 35%.[7] Pregnancy is a hypercoagulable state that can persist up to 6 to 12 weeks after delivery.[59] In addition, HF is itself a prothrombotic state because of associated endothelial dysfunction and stasis of blood. In the antepartum period, low-molecular-weight heparin or unfractionated heparin may be administered. Postpartum, warfarin may be given. Bromocriptine is associated with thromboembolic events and thus its administration should always be accompanied with anticoagulation.[7,59]

Anti-inflammatory Therapy

Pentoxifylline, which inhibits tumor necrosis factor-α, was studied in a small trial. There was significant improvement in LVEF and reduction in composite end point of poor outcomes (death, NYHA functional class III/IV, failure to improve LVEF by at least 10%) in the group treated with pentoxifylline.[60] A pilot study investigated intravenous immune globulin therapy in six PPCM patients and found significant improvement in LVEF in the treatment group.[61] Given the limited data supporting these medications in PPCM, immunosuppression and immunomodulatory therapy are not currently recommended as routine treatment.

Advanced Heart Failure Therapies

If hemodynamic stability cannot be achieved in the antepartum period, urgent delivery via caesarean section is recommended. Advanced HF therapies, including mechanical circulatory support, may need to be considered. Intra-aortic balloon pump, Impella, and extracorporeal membrane oxygenation have all been used in the treatment of PPCM patients with acute severe HF.[62,63] Durable therapies, such as bridge-to-recovery or bridge-to-LV assist device and transplant, are considered in severe cases that do adequately not respond to these therapies.[7]

Contraception

Counseling regarding future pregnancy and contraception is advised. A recent study of 177 patients with history of PPCM reported that more than 25% of sexually active women were not using contraception and one-third did not receive counseling about risks of subsequent pregnancies and contraceptive options.[64] Given increased risk of HF relapse with subsequent pregnancies and the potential teratogenicity of medications used to treat HF, unplanned future pregnancies should be avoided. Safety and efficacy must be considered when choosing a method of contraception. Combined hormonal methods including the combined oral contraceptive pill, the vaginal ring, and the transdermal patch are associated with an increased risk for thromboembolism and hypertension, and are associated with 1-year typical-use failure rate of 9%.[65,66] Long-acting reversible methods of contraception, including intrauterine devices and the subdermal implant, are preferred.[7] These methods have a 1-year typical-use failure rate of less than 1% and are considered safe for all cardiovascular conditions.[65]

Implantable Cardioverter-Defibrillator

Implantable cardioverter-defibrillator (ICD) therapy may be recommended for primary prevention of sudden cardiac death. Because many patients with PPCM may continue to recover LV function up to 12 months or longer after diagnosis, early ICD implantation may be premature.[11] PPCM experts generally agree that ICD implantation for primary prevention is recommended in patients with PPCM according to standard ICD implantation criteria, with the provision that implantation is generally deferred until completion of a minimum of 6 months of GDMT.[59,67] Wearable cardioverter-defibrillators have been studied for prevention of sudden cardiac death and may be of benefit in patients with severely reduced LVEF for the first 3 to 6 months after diagnosis.[68,69]

Long-Term Implications

Prognosis following diagnosis of PPCM is heterogeneous. Mortality has been reported to range between 0% and 19%, with only 4% mortality in the IPAC study.[11,70] Black women have increased rates of death and other major adverse events.[11,12,15] In 2013, PPCM accounted for 5% of all cardiac transplants performed in the United States.[15]

Up to 72% of women with PPCM have been reported to have improvement of LVEF to greater than or equal to 50% with medical therapy.[11] In the IPAC study, 86% of women with initial LVEF greater than or equal to 30% had recovery of LVEF to greater than or equal to 50%, compared with only 37% of women with initial LVEF less than 30%.[11] RV function, as measured by RV fractional area change, was identified as a predictor of LVEF recovery in the IPAC study.[71] Gestational hypertension and preeclampsia have been associated with increased likelihood of LV recovery.[14,21] Negative predictors of recovery include LVEF less than 30%, LV end-diastolic diameter greater than or equal to 6.0 cm, black race,[11] and clinical presentation before delivery (**Fig. 1**).[14] Most patients who have improvement in LVEF show

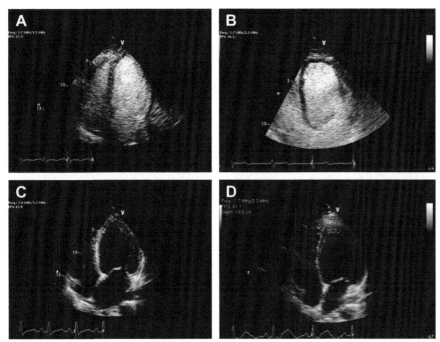

Fig. 1. Transthoracic echocardiographic images of two women with peripartum cardiomyopathy. *Top row*: Apical four-chamber images at diagnosis (*A*) and 1 year later (*B*) of a white patient with PPCM and concomitant preeclampsia with subsequent recovery of LV function. LVEF was 20%, LVEDD of 5.3 cm (normal), and RV function normal at diagnosis. LVEF was 55%, LVEDD of 4.6 cm, and RV function normal 1 year later. *Second row*: Apical four-chamber images at diagnosis (*C*) and 1 year later (*D*) of an African American patient with PPCM and no preeclampsia with lack of recovery of LV function. LVEF was 27%, LVEDD of 5.7 cm, and RV mildly dysfunctional at diagnosis. Despite maximal medical therapy, LVEF had declined to 19% and LVEDD increased to 7.0 cm 1 year later. Preeclampsia has been associated with LVEF recovery. African descent, RV involvement, and LV dilatation have been associated with poor prognosis. LVEDD, left ventricular end-diastolic diameter.

echocardiographic evidence of recovery within the first 2 to 6 months after diagnosis, although continued improvement is seen up until 1 year or even longer after diagnosis.[13,72]

Data are limited regarding the value of continuation of medical therapy after LV recovery in women with PPCM. Amos and colleagues[72] did not observe a decline in LV function after discontinuation of HF medications in a small number of patients over an average follow-up of 29 months. Patients are frequently counseled to continue medical therapy for a period of time after LV recovery, whereas some patients are counseled to continue medical therapy indefinitely because there is a small risk of HF relapse outside the setting of subsequent pregnancy.[17,73]

Several studies have reported that women with LV recovery have an approximately 20% risk of recurrent HF symptoms or decline in LV function with subsequent pregnancy and that some of these women will experience persistent LV dysfunction postpartum.[74,75] A recent single center study reported a relapse rate of 21%. None of the patients had LVEF decline to the level of their

index pregnancy, no cardiac arrests or deaths were observed, and all patients with relapse had full LV recovery with a median time to LV recovery of 1 month.[76] All but 1 of the 25 patients had fully recovered LV function before subsequent pregnancy. Other studies have reported that mortality in women with recovered LVEF and subsequent pregnancy is comparable with the general pregnant population.[74,77]

In contrast, patients who have LVEF less than 50% before subsequent pregnancies have an approximately 50% incidence of recurrent HF symptoms and up to 25% mortality.[74,75,77] Thus, subsequent pregnancy is discouraged for women with a history of PPCM and persistent LV dysfunction.[7,59] Pregnancy is also not recommended for women with severe LV dysfunction (LVEF <25%) at diagnosis, even with later recovery of LVEF.[7] Subsequent pregnancies among women with history of PPCM require multidisciplinary management with serial clinical and echocardiographic evaluation throughout the peripartum period.[70]

Because of reports of HF relapse outside the setting of subsequent pregnancy, patients with history of PPCM should optimally be evaluated with serial clinical examinations and echocardiograms for an extended period of time, perhaps indefinitely. No very-long-term studies of the natural history of patients with PPCM have been published, so long-term risks for women with this disease remain unknown. Other forms of cardiovascular disease related to pregnancy, including gestational hypertension and preeclampsia, have been shown to increase risk for the development of cardiovascular disease in women,[78] so it seems reasonable to consider that patients with history of PPCM may have increased risk for recurrent HF or other forms of cardiovascular disease as they age.

FUTURE DIRECTIONS

Although substantial progress has been made over the past decade regarding the pathophysiology, management, and natural history of PPCM, many questions remain unanswered. The likely complex interaction between genetic and environmental factors that lead to the development of PPCM has not yet been completely elucidated. Optimal treatment strategies, regarding type and duration of therapy, are not well-defined. Accurate prognostication regarding LV recovery, risk for relapse with subsequent pregnancy, and risk for long-term cardiovascular events is lacking. Large-scale prospective studies are warranted to answer these important questions.

REFERENCES

1. Meigs C. Letter XXXVIII. In: Females and their diseases: a series of letters to his class. Philadelphia: Lea and Blanchard; 1848. p. 505–6.
2. Hull E, Hafkesbring E. "Toxic" postpartum heart disease. New Orleans Med Surg J 1937;89:550–7.
3. Gouley B, McMillan T, Bellet S. Idiopathic myocardial degeneration associated with pregnancy and especially the puerperium. Am J Med Sci 1937;19: 185–99.
4. Meadows R. Idiopathic myocardial failure in the last trimester of pregnancy and the puerperium. Circulation 1957;15:903–14.
5. Demakis JG, Rahimtoola SH. Peripartum cardiomyopathy. Circulation 1971;44(5):964–8.
6. Pearson GD, Veille JC, Rahimtoola S, et al. Peripartum cardiomyopathy: National Heart, Lung, and Blood Institute and Office of Rare Diseases (National Institutes of Health) workshop recommendations and review. JAMA 2000;283(9):1183–8.
7. Sliwa K, Hilfiker-Kleiner D, Petrie MC, et al. Current state of knowledge on aetiology, diagnosis, management, and therapy of peripartum cardiomyopathy: a position statement from the Heart Failure Association of the European Society of Cardiology Working Group on peripartum cardiomyopathy. Eur J Heart Fail 2010;12(8):767–78.
8. Fett JD, Christie LG, Carraway RD, et al. Five-year prospective study of the incidence and prognosis of peripartum cardiomyopathy at a single institution. Mayo Clin Proc 2005;80(12):1602–6.
9. Kamiya CA, Kitakaze M, Ishibashi-Ueda H, et al. Different characteristics of peripartum cardiomyopathy between patients complicated with and without hypertensive disorders. Results from the Japanese Nationwide survey of peripartum cardiomyopathy. Circ J 2011;75(8):1975–81.
10. Kolte D, Khera S, Aronow WS, et al. Temporal trends in incidence and outcomes of peripartum cardiomyopathy in the United States: a nationwide population-based study. J Am Heart Assoc 2014; 3(3):e001056.
11. McNamara DM, Elkayam U, Alharethi R, et al. Clinical outcomes for peripartum cardiomyopathy in North America: results of the IPAC Study (Investigations of Pregnancy-Associated Cardiomyopathy). J Am Coll Cardiol 2015;66(8):905–14.
12. Irizarry OC, Levine LD, Lewey J, et al. Comparison of clinical characteristics and outcomes of peripartum cardiomyopathy between African American and non-African American women. JAMA Cardiol 2017;2(11):1256–60.
13. Elkayam U, Akhter MW, Singh H, et al. Pregnancy-associated cardiomyopathy: clinical characteristics and a comparison between early and late presentation. Circulation 2005;111(16):2050–5.
14. Safirstein JG, Ro AS, Grandhi S, et al. Predictors of left ventricular recovery in a cohort of peripartum cardiomyopathy patients recruited via the internet. Int J Cardiol 2012;154(1):27–31.
15. Bello N, Rendon IS, Arany Z. The relationship between pre-eclampsia and peripartum cardiomyopathy: a systematic review and meta-analysis. J Am Coll Cardiol 2013;62(18):1715–23.
16. Ntusi NB, Mayosi BM. Aetiology and risk factors of peripartum cardiomyopathy: a systematic review. Int J Cardiol 2009;131(2):168–79.
17. Goland S, Modi K, Bitar F, et al. Clinical profile and predictors of complications in peripartum cardiomyopathy. J Card Fail 2009;15(8):645–50.
18. Blauwet LA, Cooper LT. Diagnosis and management of peripartum cardiomyopathy. Heart 2011;97(23): 1970–81.
19. Sliwa K, Mebazaa A, Hilfiker-Kleiner D, et al. Clinical characteristics of patients from the worldwide registry on peripartum cardiomyopathy (PPCM): EURObservational Research Programme in conjunction with the Heart Failure Association of the European Society of Cardiology Study Group on PPCM. Eur J Heart Fail 2017;19(9):1131–41.

20. Forster O, Hilfiker-Kleiner D, Ansari AA, et al. Reversal of IFN-gamma, oxLDL and prolactin serum levels correlate with clinical improvement in patients with peripartum cardiomyopathy. Eur J Heart Fail 2008;10(9):861–8.

21. Lindley KJ, Conner SN, Cahill AG, et al. Impact of preeclampsia on clinical and functional outcomes in women with peripartum cardiomyopathy. Circ Heart Fail 2017;10(6) [pii:e003797].

22. Haghikia A, Rontgen P, Vogel-Claussen J, et al. Prognostic implication of right ventricular involvement in peripartum cardiomyopathy: a cardiovascular magnetic resonance study. ESC Heart Fail 2015; 2(4):139–49.

23. Mouquet F, Lions C, de Groote P, et al. Characterisation of peripartum cardiomyopathy by cardiac magnetic resonance imaging. Eur Radiol 2008;18(12): 2765–9.

24. Renz DM, Rottgen R, Habedank D, et al. New insights into peripartum cardiomyopathy using cardiac magnetic resonance imaging. Rofo 2011; 183(9):834–41.

25. Arora NP, Mohamad T, Mahajan N, et al. Cardiac magnetic resonance imaging in peripartum cardiomyopathy. Am J Med Sci 2014;347(2): 112–7.

26. Marmursztejn J, Vignaux O, Goffinet F, et al. Delayed-enhanced cardiac magnetic resonance imaging features in peripartum cardiomyopathy. Int J Cardiol 2009;137:e63–4.

27. Pearl W. Familial occurrence of peripartum cardiomyopathy. Am Heart J 1995;129(2):421–2.

28. Fett JD, Sundstrom BJ, Etta King M, et al. Mother-daughter peripartum cardiomyopathy. Int J Cardiol 2002;86(2–3):331–2.

29. Kamiya CA, Yoshimatsu J, Ikeda T. Peripartum cardiomyopathy from a genetic perspective. Circ J 2016;80(8):1684–8.

30. Ware JS, Li J, Mazaika E, et al. Shared genetic predisposition in peripartum and dilated cardiomyopathies. N Engl J Med 2016;374(3):233–41.

31. van Spaendonck-Zwarts KY, Posafalvi A, van den Berg MP, et al. Titin gene mutations are common in families with both peripartum cardiomyopathy and dilated cardiomyopathy. Eur Heart J 2014;35(32): 2165–73.

32. Sheppard R, Hsich E, Damp J, et al. GNB3 C825T polymorphism and myocardial recovery in peripartum cardiomyopathy: results of the multicenter investigations of pregnancy-associated cardiomyopathy study. Circ Heart Fail 2016;9(3): e002683.

33. Xia G, Zheng X, Yao X, et al. Expression of programmed cell death-1 and its ligand B7 homolog 1 in peripheral blood lymphocytes from patients with peripartum cardiomyopathy. Clin Cardiol 2017; 40(5):307–13.

34. Sayama S, Nagamatsu T, Schust DJ, et al. Human decidual macrophages suppress IFN-gamma production by T cells through costimulatory B7-H1: PD-1 signaling in early pregnancy. J Reprod Immunol 2013;100(2):109–17.

35. Xia G, Sun X, Zheng X, et al. Decreased expression of programmed death 1 on peripheral blood lymphocytes disrupts immune homeostasis in peripartum cardiomyopathy. Int J Cardiol 2016;223:842–7.

36. McTiernan CF, Morel P, Cooper LT, et al. Circulating T-cell subsets, monocytes, and natural killer cells in peripartum cardiomyopathy: results from the Multicenter IPAC Study. J Card Fail 2018;24(1):33–42.

37. Ansari AA, Fett JD, Carraway RE, et al. Autoimmune mechanisms as the basis for human peripartum cardiomyopathy. Clin Rev Allergy Immunol 2002;23(3): 301–24.

38. Bultmann BD, Klingel K, Nabauer M, et al. High prevalence of viral genomes and inflammation in peripartum cardiomyopathy. Am J Obstet Gynecol 2005;193(2):363–5.

39. Patten IS, Rana S, Shahul S, et al. Cardiac angiogenic imbalance leads to peripartum cardiomyopathy. Nature 2012;485(7398):333–8.

40. Bello NA, Arany Z. Molecular mechanisms of peripartum cardiomyopathy: a vascular/hormonal hypothesis. Trends Cardiovasc Med 2015;25(6): 499–504.

41. Goland S, Weinstein JM, Zalik A, et al. Angiogenic imbalance and residual myocardial injury in recovered peripartum cardiomyopathy patients. Circ Heart Fail 2016;9(11) [pii:e003349].

42. Hilfiker-Kleiner D, Kaminski K, Podewski E, et al. A cathepsin D-cleaved 16 kDa form of prolactin mediates postpartum cardiomyopathy. Cell 2007; 128(3):589–600.

43. Mebazaa A, Seronde MF, Gayat E, et al. Imbalanced angiogenesis in peripartum cardiomyopathy. Diagnostic value of placenta growth factor. Circ J 2017; 81(11):1654–61.

44. Damp J, Givertz MM, Semigran M, et al. Relaxin-2 and Soluble Flt1 levels in peripartum cardiomyopathy: results of the multicenter IPAC study. JACC Heart Fail 2016;4(5):380–8.

45. Noori M, Donald AE, Angelakopoulou A, et al. Prospective study of placental angiogenic factors and maternal vascular function before and after preeclampsia and gestational hypertension. Circulation 2010;122(5):478–87.

46. Tuzcu ZB, Asicioglu E, Sunbul M, et al. Circulating endothelial cell number and markers of endothelial dysfunction in previously preeclamptic women. Am J Obstet Gynecol 2015;213(4):533.e1-7.

47. Petrozella L, Mahendroo M, Timmons B, et al. Endothelial microparticles and the antiangiogenic state in preeclampsia and the postpartum period. Am J Obstet Gynecol 2012;207(2):140.e20-6.

48. Desplantie O, Tremblay-Gravel M, Avram R, et al. The medical treatment of new-onset peripartum cardiomyopathy: a systematic review of prospective studies. Can J Cardiol 2015;31(12):1421–6.

49. Frishman WH, Elkayam U, Aronow WS. Cardiovascular drugs in pregnancy. Cardiol Clin 2012;30(3): 463–91.

50. Lactmed. Available at: https://toxnet.nlm.nih.gov/newtoxnet/lactmed.htm. Accessed September 16, 2017.

51. Haghikia A, Tongers J, Berliner D, et al. Early ivabradine treatment in patients with acute peripartum cardiomyopathy: subanalysis of the German PPCM registry. Int J Cardiol 2016;216:165–7.

52. Demir S, Tufenk M, Karakaya Z, et al. The treatment of heart failure-related symptoms with ivabradine in a case with peripartum cardiomyopathy. Int Cardiovasc Res J 2013;7(1):33–6.

53. Gaddipati VC, Patel AA, Cohen AJ. The use of a novel heart failure agent in the treatment of pregnancy-associated cardiomyopathy. Case Rep Cardiol 2017;2017:9561405.

54. Hubers SA, Brown NJ. Combined angiotensin receptor antagonism and neprilysin inhibition. Circulation 2016;133(11):1115–24.

55. Sag S, Coskun H, Baran I, et al. Inappropriate sinus tachycardia-induced cardiomyopathy during pregnancy and successful treatment with ivabradine. Anatol J Cardiol 2016;16(3):212–3.

56. Sliwa K, Blauwet L, Tibazarwa K, et al. Evaluation of bromocriptine in the treatment of acute severe peripartum cardiomyopathy: a proof-of-concept pilot study. Circulation 2010;121(13):1465–73.

57. Haghikia A, Podewski E, Libhaber E, et al. Phenotyping and outcome on contemporary management in a German cohort of patients with peripartum cardiomyopathy. Basic Res Cardiol 2013;108(4):366.

58. Hilfiker-Kleiner D, Haghikia A, Berliner D, et al. Bromocriptine for the treatment of peripartum cardiomyopathy: a multicentre randomized study. Eur Heart J 2017;38(35):2671–9.

59. European Society of Gynecology (ESG), Association for European Paediatric Cardiology (AEPC), German Society for Gender Medicine (DGesGM), et al. ESC Guidelines on the management of cardiovascular diseases during pregnancy: the Task Force on the Management of Cardiovascular Diseases during Pregnancy of the European Society of Cardiology (ESC). Eur Heart J 2011;32(24):3147–97.

60. Sliwa K, Skudicky D, Candy G, et al. The addition of pentoxifylline to conventional therapy improves outcome in patients with peripartum cardiomyopathy. Eur J Heart Fail 2002;4(3):305–9.

61. Bozkurt B, Villanueva FS, Holubkov R, et al. Intravenous immune globulin in the therapy of peripartum cardiomyopathy. J Am Coll Cardiol 1999;34(1): 177–80.

62. Bouabdallaoui N, Demondion P, Leprince P, et al. Short-term mechanical circulatory support for cardiogenic shock in severe peripartum cardiomyopathy: La Pitie-Salpetriere experience. Interact Cardiovasc Thorac Surg 2017;25(1):52–6.

63. Gevaert S, Van Belleghem Y, Bouchez S, et al. Acute and critically ill peripartum cardiomyopathy and 'bridge to' therapeutic options: a single center experience with intra-aortic balloon pump, extra corporeal membrane oxygenation and continuous-flow left ventricular assist devices. Crit Care 2011;15(2):R93.

64. Rosman L, Salmoirago-Blotcher E, Wuensch KL, et al. Contraception and reproductive counseling in women with peripartum cardiomyopathy. Contraception 2017;96(1):36–40.

65. Centers for Disease Control and Prevention. U.S. Selected practice recommendations for contraceptive use. Morbidity Mortality Weekly Rep 2013;62(5):1–60.

66. Tepper NK, Paulen ME, Marchbanks PA, et al. Safety of contraceptive use among women with peripartum cardiomyopathy: a systematic review. Contraception 2010;82(1):95–101.

67. Russo AM, Stainback RF, Bailey SR, et al. ACCF/HRS/AHA/ASE/HFSA/SCAI/SCCT/SCMR 2013 appropriate use criteria for implantable cardioverter-defibrillators and cardiac resynchronization therapy: a report of the American College of Cardiology Foundation appropriate use criteria task force, Heart Rhythm Society, American Heart Association, American Society of Echocardiography, Heart Failure Society of America, Society for Cardiovascular Angiography and Interventions, Society of Cardiovascular Computed Tomography, and Society for Cardiovascular Magnetic Resonance. Heart Rhythm 2013; 10(4):e11–58.

68. Duncker D, Westenfeld R, Konrad T, et al. Risk for life-threatening arrhythmia in newly diagnosed peripartum cardiomyopathy with low ejection fraction: a German multi-centre analysis. Clin Res Cardiol 2017;106(8):582–9.

69. Duncker D, Haghikia A, Konig T, et al. Risk for ventricular fibrillation in peripartum cardiomyopathy with severely reduced left ventricular function-value of the wearable cardioverter/defibrillator. Eur J Heart Fail 2014;16(12):1331–6.

70. Elkayam U. Clinical characteristics of peripartum cardiomyopathy in the United States: diagnosis, prognosis, and management. J Am Coll Cardiol 2011;58(7):659–70.

71. Blauwet LA, Delgado-Montero A, Ryo K, et al. Right ventricular function in peripartum cardiomyopathy at presentation is associated with subsequent left ventricular recovery and clinical outcomes. Circ Heart Fail 2016;9(5) [pii:e002756].

72. Amos AM, Jaber WA, Russell SD. Improved outcomes in peripartum cardiomyopathy with contemporary. Am Heart J 2006;152(3):509–13.

73. Mahowald MK, Davis M. Case series: spontaneous relapse after recovery from peripartum cardiomyopathy. Clin Med Insights Case Rep 2017;10. 1179547617749227.

74. Elkayam U, Tummala PP, Rao K, et al. Maternal and fetal outcomes of subsequent pregnancies in women with peripartum cardiomyopathy. N Engl J Med 2001;344(21):1567–71.

75. Fett JD, Fristoe KL, Welsh SN. Risk of heart failure relapse in subsequent pregnancy among peripartum cardiomyopathy mothers. Int J Gynaecol Obstet 2010;109(1):34–6.

76. Codsi E, Rose CH, Blauwet LA. Subsequent pregnancy outcomes in patients with peripartum cardiomyopathy. Obstet Gynecol 2018;131(2):322–7.

77. Hilfiker-Kleiner D, Haghikia A, Masuko D, et al. Outcome of subsequent pregnancies in patients with a history of peripartum cardiomyopathy. Eur J Heart Fail 2017;19(12):1723–8.

78. Mosca L, Benjamin EJ, Berra K, et al. Effectiveness-based guidelines for the prevention of cardiovascular disease in women—2011 update: a guideline from the American Heart Association. J Am Coll Cardiol 2011;57(12):1404–23.

Stress-Induced Cardiomyopathy

Lili Zhang, MD, MS[a], Ileana L. Piña, MD, MPH[b],*

KEYWORDS

- Apical ballooning syndrome • Clinical features • Outcomes • Stress induced cardiomyopathy
- Takotsubo syndrome

KEY POINTS

- Stress-induced cardiomyopathy is characterized by reversible myocardial injury with distinctive regional wall motion abnormalities of the left ventricle.
- It has a strong predilection for women and postmenopausal women.
- Patients often present with chest pain, ST-segment changes on electrocardiogram, and elevated cardiac enzyme levels, but an absence of obstructive coronary artery disease.
- Patients can be frequently complicated by acute heart failure, cardiogenic shock, arrhythmia, left ventricular outflow tract obstruction and ventricular thrombi, among others.
- Supportive measures are the mainstay of management. The prognosis of this condition is not benign with substantial mortality and a high recurrence rate.

INTRODUCTION

Stress-induced cardiomyopathy (SIC), also called Takotsubo cardiomyopathy, left ventricular apical ballooning syndrome, or broken heart syndrome, is characterized by acute myocardial injury with distinctive regional contraction failure of the left ventricle (LV), usually precipitated by a significant emotional or physical stressor. Patients are predominantly women, especially postmenopausal women.[1] Patients often present with chest pain, ST-segment changes on the electrocardiogram (ECG), and elevated cardiac enzyme levels consistent with acute coronary syndrome (ACS). However, the LV dysfunction is independent of epicardial coronary artery obstruction and is typically completely reversible.[2,3] Apical ballooning pattern, first described and published in Japan in 1990, is present in majority of the patients.[4,5]

Epidemiology

SIC is an uncommon condition in the general population. According to the Nationwide Inpatient Sample database, 6837 patients were diagnosed with SIC among 33,506,402 hospitalizations in the United States in 2008. The prevalence of SIC in this study was approximately 0.02%.[5] In comparison, the number of patients discharged with ACS was 883,000 in 2001.[6] It was also found that the incidence of SIC has increased from 2006 (0.11 per 100,000 person-years) to 2012 (1.98 per 100,000 person-years), most likely owing to the increasing recognition of the syndrome.[7] Across multiple series, 1% to 2% of all patients who had suspected ACS have been identified as having SIC.[4,8–11] From a statistical analysis of reported case series in the literature, patients were found to be typically Asian (57.2%) or Caucasian (40%) and only 2.8% of patients were with of another race/ethnicity.[12]

Disclosure Statement: The authors have nothing to disclose.
a Division of Cardiology, Montefiore Medical Center, 111 East 210th Street, Bronx, NY 10467, USA; b Division of Cardiology, Montefiore Medical Center, Albert Einstein College of Medicine, 1825 Eastchester Road, 2nd Floor Cardiology, Bronx, NY 10467, USA
* Corresponding author.
E-mail address: ilpina@montefiore.org

Heart Failure Clin 15 (2019) 41–53
https://doi.org/10.1016/j.hfc.2018.08.005
1551-7136/19/© 2018 Elsevier Inc. All rights reserved.

heartfailure.theclinics.com

Numerous studies have reported a preponderance of SIC among postmenopausal women.[2,3,5,13,14] Based on the International Takotsubo Registry, a consortium of 26 centers from Europe and the United States, of 1750 patients enrolled, 89.8% were women and 79.1% were women older than 50 years of age.[13] According to the Nationwide Inpatient Sample database, patients of SIC aged from 50 to 79 years were 72.1%, compared with 17.6% of patients with SIC aged 80 years or older and 10.4% of patients aged from 18 to 49 years. Women older than 55 years of age had a 4.8 times higher odds of developing SIC when compared with women younger than 55 years of age.[5] The incidence of SIC increased over the years for all age groups in women, but the increase in the age group of 45 to 84 years was much higher than the patients of other age groups. In contrast, the yearly incidence remained low and relatively stable in men.[7] A decrease in estrogen levels after menopause and greater prevalence of microvascular abnormalities may predispose older women to SIC.[15]

Multiple risk factors of SIC have been reported. The National Inpatient Sample database suggested that smoking, alcohol abuse, anxiety states, and hyperlipidemia were commonly associated with SIC.[5] The International Takotsubo Registry reported that physical triggers (such as acute respiratory failure, postoperative stress, fracture, central nervous system conditions, and infection) were more common than emotional triggers (such as grief, panic, fear, anxiety, interpersonal conflict, and anger; 36% vs 27.7%), although 28.5% of patients had no clear triggers. As compared with ACS, rates of neurologic or psychiatric disorders were higher in patients with SIC (55.8% vs 25.7%).[13]

Pathophysiology

Although the cause of SIC remains unknown, several theories have been proposed and are under investigation.[16,17] The hypothesis of excess catecholamine concentration resulting in catecholamine-induced myocardial stunning is the most widely accepted.[18] It is supported by the temporal relationship between a stressful event and the onset of symptoms and the cases triggered by iatrogenic catecholamine administration.[19] The neurohormonal stimulation can lead to acute myocardial dysfunction through "brain–heart interaction." The mechanisms of ventricular dysfunction include multivessel/microvascular vasospasm, endothelial dysfunction, direct catecholamine-mediated myocardial stunning, and increased ventricular afterload.[18]

Microvascular dysfunction has been advocated as a pathophysiologic hypothesis underlying SIC.[20] It has a female preponderance and has been detected in up to 50% of women presenting with angina. Many studies have investigated microvascular dysfunction in SIC using various techniques.[21–24] Although mostly with small sample size, these studies consistently demonstrated acute and transient involvement of microvascular dysfunction in patients with SIC. Nuclear imaging techniques, such as single-photon emission computed tomography (SPECT) and positron emission tomography (PET), found disturbance of cardiac sympathetic innervation, fatty acid and glucose metabolism in patients with SIC. These abnormalities were often more profound and more persistent than myocardial perfusion abnormalities.[24–27] The presence of this "inverse perfusion–metabolism mismatch" suggests diffuse microvascular abnormalities.

It needs to kept in mind that SIC and coronary artery disease (CAD) may not be mutually exclusive. Case series of patients with SIC with LV wall motion abnormalities of Takotsubo pattern were reported to have bystander CAD, even obstructive CAD.[28,29] A less popular hypothesis of pathogenesis of SIC is spontaneously aborted myocardial infarction resulting from an acute atherosclerotic event with rapid and complete lysis of the thrombus,[30,31] although there are no solid data to support this hypothesis.

Clinical Presentation

Diagnosis

Diagnosis criteria Patients with SIC commonly present with substernal chest pain. ECG changes include ST-segment elevation, T-wave inversion, QT-interval prolongation, abnormal Q-waves or nonspecific abnormalities. Increases in cardiac biomarkers are typically less pronounced than in ACS and coronary angiography does not reveal obstructive CAD or plaque rupture corresponding to the wall motion abnormalities seen in this condition. There are multiple diagnostic criteria of SIC published so far (**Box 1**) and the most widely used are the modified Mayo clinic criteria.[32–35] However, owing to the increasing awareness of SIC, diversity of the clinical presentation, and rapidly expanding literature, the criteria based on clinical features only were thought to be outmoded.[36,37] Diagnosis of SIC cases overlapping CAD or mimicking myocarditis or pheochromocytoma is often debatable. The use of noninvasive imaging tools for the diagnosis of SIC has been studied with great interest. Cardiovascular magnetic resonance (CMR) shows some

---

Box 1
Different diagnostic criteria for stress-induced cardiomyopathy

Modified Mayo Clinic[32]

1. Transient hypokinesis, akinesis, or dyskinesis of the left ventricular midsegments with or without apical involvement; the regional wall motion abnormalities extend beyond a single epicardial vascular distribution; a stressful trigger is often, but not always present.[a]

2. Absence of obstructive coronary disease or angiographic evidence of acute plaque rupture.[b]

3. New electrocardiographic abnormalities (either ST-segment elevation and/or T-wave inversion) or modest elevation in cardiac troponin.

4. Absence of pheochromocytoma or myocarditis.

> In both of these circumstances, the diagnosis of apical ballooning syndrome (ABS) should be made with caution, and a clear stressful precipitating trigger must be sought.

Japanese Criteria[33]

1. Definition

> Takotsubo (ampulla) cardiomyopathy is a disease exhibiting an acute left ventricular apical ballooning of unknown cause.

> In this disease, the left ventricle takes on the shape of a "Takotsubo" (Japanese octopus trap). There is nearly complete resolution of the apical akinesis in the majority of the patients within 1 month. The contraction abnormality occurs mainly in the left ventricle, but involvement of the right ventricle is observed in some cases. A dynamic obstruction of the left ventricular outflow tract (pressure gradient difference, acceleration of blood flow, or systolic cardiac murmurs) is also observed.

> Note: There are patients, such as cerebrovascular patients, who have an apical systolic ballooning similar to that in Takotsubo cardiomyopathy, but with a known cause. Such patients are diagnosed as "cerebrovascular disease with Takotsubo-like myocardial dysfunction" and are differentiated from idiopathic cases.

2. References for diagnosis

   A. Symptoms: Chest pain and dyspnea similar to those in acute coronary syndrome. Takotsubo cardiomyopathy can occur without symptoms.

   B. Triggers: Emotional or physical stress may trigger Takotsubo cardiomyopathy, but it can also occur without any apparent trigger.

   C. Age and gender difference: Known tendency to increase in the elderly, particularly females.

   D. Ventricular morphology: Apical ballooning and its rapid improvement in the ventriculogram and echocardiogram.

   E. Electrocardiogram: ST-segment elevations might be observed immediately after the onset. Thereafter, in a typical case, the T-wave becomes progressively more negative in multiple leads and the QT interval prolongs. These changes improve gradually, but a negative T wave may continue for several months. During the acute stage, abnormal Q waves and changes in the QRS voltage might be observed.

   F. Cardiac biomarkers: In a typical case, there are only modest increases in serum levels of cardiac enzymes and troponin.

   G. Myocardial radionuclear study: Abnormal findings in myocardial scintigraphy are observed in some cases.

   H. Prognosis: The majority of the patients recover rapidly, but some patients suffer pulmonary edema and other sequelae or death.

3. Exclusion criteria

> The following lesions and abnormalities from other diseases must be excluded in the diagnosis of Takotsubo (ampulla) cardiomyopathy.

   A. Significant organic stenosis or spasm of a coronary artery. In particular, acute myocardial infarction owing to a lesion of the anterior descending branch of the left coronary artery, which perfuses an extensive territory including the left ventricular apex (an urgent coronary angiogram is desirable for imaging during the acute stage, but coronary angiography is also necessary during the chronic stage to confirm the presence or absence of a significant stenotic lesion or a lesion involved in the abnormal pattern of ventricular contraction).

B. Cerebrovascular disease

C. Pheochromocytoma

D. Viral or idiopathic myocarditis

Note: For the exclusion of coronary artery lesions, coronary angiography is required. Takotsubo-like myocardial dysfunction could occur with diseases such as cerebrovascular disease and pheochromocytoma.

Takotsubo Italian Network Investigators criteria[34]

1. Typical transient left ventricular wall motion abnormalities extending beyond a single epicardial vascular distribution with complete functional normalization within 6 weeks.

2. Absence of potentially culprit coronary stenosis, or angiographic evidence of acute plaque rupture, dissection, thrombosis or spasm.[c]

3. New and dynamic ST-segment abnormalities or T-wave inversion as well as new onset of transient or permanent left bundle branch block.

4. Mild increase in myocardial injury markers (creatine kinase-MB value of <50 U/L).

5. Clinical and/or instrumental exclusion of myocarditis.

6. Postmenopausal woman (optional).[d]

7. Antecedent stressful event (optional).[d]

European Heart Failure Association Diagnostic Criteria[2]

1. Transient regional wall motion abnormalities of left ventricular or right ventricular myocardium, which are frequently, but not always, preceded by a stressful trigger (emotional or physical).

2. The regional wall motion abnormalities usually[e] extend beyond a single epicardial vascular distribution, and often result in circumferential dysfunction of the ventricular segments involved.

3. The absence of culprit atherosclerotic coronary artery disease including acute plaque rupture, thrombus formation, and coronary dissection or other pathologic conditions to explain the pattern of temporary left ventricular dysfunction observed (eg, hypertrophic cardiomyopathy, viral myocarditis).

4. New and reversible electrocardiography abnormalities (ST-segment elevation, ST depression, left bundle branch block,[f] T-wave inversion, and/or QTc prolongation) during the acute phase (3 months).

5. Significantly elevated serum natriuretic peptide (B-type natriuretic peptide or *N*-terminal pro B-type natriuretic peptide) during the acute phase.

6. Positive but relatively small elevation in cardiac troponin measured with a conventional assay (ie, disparity between the troponin level and the amount of dysfunctional myocardium present).[g]

7. Recovery of ventricular systolic function on cardiac imaging at follow-up (3–6 months).[h]

Cardiovascular Magnetic Resonance Criteria[35]

1. Severe LV dysfunction in a noncoronary regional distribution pattern.

2. Myocardial edema colocated with the regional wall motion abnormality (edema should be verified by a quantitative signal intensity analysis, best by calculating the signal intensity ratio between myocardium and skeletal muscle [T2 signal intensity ratio]; a cutoff value of ≥ 1.9 should be used to define edema).

3. Absence of high-signal areas in late gadolinium enhancement images (a cutoff value of >5 standard deviations should be used to define significance).

4. Increased early myocardial gadolinium uptake (increased uptake is defined by an early gadolinium enhancement ratio of ≥ 4.0 [optimal cutoff values may vary between scanners]).

   The confirmative criterion (with >4-week follow-up) for all diagnostic criteria is complete or near-complete resolution.

[a] There are rare exceptions to these criteria, such as those patients in whom the regional wall motion abnormality is limited to a single coronary territory.

[b] It is possible that a patient with obstructive coronary atherosclerosis may also develop ABS. However, this is very rare in our experience and in the published literature, perhaps because such cases are misdiagnosed as an acute coronary syndrome.

[c] Coronary angiography should be performed as soon as possible (ideally within 48 hours of admission).

[d] Optional diagnostic criteria are not mandatory, but when positive they increase the likelihood of Takotsubo syndrome diagnosis.

[e] Acute, reversible dysfunction of a single coronary territory has been reported.

[f] Left bundle branch block may be permanent after Takotsubo syndrome, but should also alert clinicians to exclude other cardiomyopathies. T-wave changes and QTc prolongation may take many weeks to months to normalize after recovery of left ventricular function.

[g] Troponin-negative cases have been reported, but are atypical.

[h] Small apical infarcts have been reported. Bystander subendocardial infarcts have been reported, involving a small proportion of the acutely dysfunctional myocardium. These infarcts are insufficient to explain the acute regional wall motion abnormality observed.

promise in this regard. The most recently published CMR criteria were developed based on a prospective study conducted at 7 tertiary care centers in Europe and North America among 256 patients with SIC.[35] The criteria included tissue characterization techniques, such as quantitative signal intensity analysis, early and late gadolinium enhancement (LGE). This set of criteria can provide more objective guidance in diagnosing SIC compared with traditional clinical features, especially for challenging cases.

Differential diagnosis The differential diagnosis between SIC and ACS is challenging. In the acute phase, the clinical presentation, ECG findings, and biomarker profiles of these 2 conditions are often similar. Although an absence of obstructive CAD is a diagnostic criterion of SIC, they are not mutually exclusive. Owing to the older age of population with SIC, nonparticipant obstructive CAD may be seen in patients with SIC.[28,29] In this scenario, careful consideration is required to make the diagnosis because of its impact on subsequent treatment. In addition, in real-world clinical practice, a substantial proportion of patients with suspected SIC did not undergo coronary evaluation to exclude ACS, suggesting that the coronary angiogram has been underused in the diagnosis of SIC.[38] Many studies have investigated the differentiation between SIC and ACS from clinical presentations, ECG, and biomarkers to noninvasive imaging (**Table 1**).[13,39–44]

Acute myocarditis can also mimic SIC owing to their similar clinical presentations. In some cases, acute myocarditis may present with regional LV wall motion abnormalities similar to those of typical SIC cases.[45] CMR may be helpful in this setting because acute myocarditis is characterized by LGE of various patterns, whereas LGE is generally absent in patients with SIC.[35]

Sex differences in clinical presentation
Women and men have some discrepancies in clinical profiles of SIC.[15] In a German registry of 324 patients with SIC (296 women and 28 men), physical stress was more frequent in men, whereas more women experienced emotional stress or no stress. Fewer women were admitted in cardiogenic shock and/or after out-of-hospital cardiac arrest, and the cardiac troponin level was lower. The QTc interval was longer in women than in men on the day of admission. The clinical complications during the acute course were comparable in both groups.[1] In 368 patients with SIC (84 male, 284 female) from the Tokyo cardiac care unit (CCU) Network database, no significant differences was found in apical ballooning type, median ejection fraction by echocardiography, serious ventricular arrhythmias, or cardiovascular death between male and female patients. However, severe pump failure and cardiopulmonary supportive therapies were found more commonly in male patients. Male gender was an independent predictor of adverse composite cardiac events, including cardiovascular death, severe pump failure, and serious ventricular arrhythmia.[46] According to the National Inpatient Sample database, male patients with SIC had higher incidence of underlying critical illnesses (36.6% vs 26.8%) and higher in-hospital mortality (8.4% vs 3.6%) than their female counterparts.[47] In a retrospective study consisting of 114 patients with SIC, all-cause mortality of male patients revealed to be 2.6 times higher than that for female patients over a 5-year follow-up period. Most males died of noncardiac causes, such as progressive cancer disease and sepsis. Nevertheless, cardiac cause of death and cardiovascular events were similar in male and female patients.[48]

Racial and ethnic differences in clinical presentation
Current data on racial differences of SIC are inconsistent, but growing evidence suggests racial disparities exist in patients with SIC. In a series of 206 patients with SIC from different racial and ethnic backgrounds, African American patients were older and had a longer duration of stay at the index

Table 1
Differences between stress-induced cardiomyopathy and acute myocardial infarction

	Stress-Induced Cardiomyopathy	Acute Myocardial Infarction
Clinical presentation	• Postmenopausal women predominant • Physical or emotional stress • History of neurologic or psychiatric disorder • LV outflow tract obstruction • LV mural thrombosis	• Male predominant • Coronary artery disease risk factors
Electrocardiogram	• PR-segment depression • Maximum ST-segment elevation of ≤0.2 mV • No reciprocal changes in inferior leads • QT prolongation	• ST segment elevation • ST segment depression • T wave inversion • Abnormal Q wave
Coronary angiogram	• No or mild coronary artery disease • Extent and location of coronary artery disease not matching the territory of LV wall motion abnormalities • Increased LV end-diastolic pressure	• Critical coronary obstruction or evidence of acute plaque rupture • LV wall motion abnormalities matching the territory of coronary artery disease
Biomarkers	• Mildly elevated troponin and CK • High BNP levels	• High troponin and CK levels • Variable BNP levels
Imaging	• Apical and/or midventricular hypokinesis and basal hyperkinesis • LVEF and wall motion abnormalities recover within 4–8 wk for most patients • CMR: transmural myocardial edema and absence of late gadolinium enhancement	• Echocardiography: LV recovery depending on revascularization and reverse remodeling • CMR: Presence of late gadolinium enhancement
Treatment	• Supportive	• Percutaneous cutaneous intervention • Aspirin, beta-blocker and statin

Abbreviations: BNP, B-type natriuretic peptide; CK, creatine kinase; CMR, cardiovascular magnetic resonance; LV, left ventricle; LVEF, left ventricular ejection fraction.

event. Hispanics had a higher prevalence of both diabetes mellitus and hyperlipidemia. Caucasians had the highest prevalence of emotional stress as the triggering event. African Americans had a more complicated clinical course evidenced by lower initial and follow-up LV ejection fraction (LVEF), and higher incidences of LV thrombus, acute respiratory failure requiring mechanical ventilation, acute heart failure, and in-hospital mortality during the index event.[49] In 800 inpatient admissions from 6 states in the United States, Asian and African American patients had a significantly higher risk of death than Caucasian patients (odds ratios, 15.1 and 2.9, respectively), although there was no significant mortality difference between white and Hispanic patients.[50] In addition, African American patients more frequently presented with diffuse T-wave inversions and a more prolonged QTc, whereas non-African American patients more often presented with ST

depression.[51] However, the National Inpatient Sample database showed that race was not associated with in-hospital death in a multivariable adjusted analysis.[47]

Complications

Left ventricular dysfunction Acute heart failure is the most common complication of SIC.[2] According to the National Inpatient Sample database, the incidence of acute heart failure was 31.1% with a mortality rate of 5%. About 5% of patients developed cardiogenic shock. An intraaortic balloon pump was used in approximately 3% of cases and these patients had high mortality rate (18.5%).[47] In 118 consecutive patients with SIC, the incidence of acute heart failure was 45%, in which 38% of patients required an inotrope, 17% of patients required intraaortic balloon pump support, and 28% of patients required mechanical ventilation.[52] In the International Takotsubo

Registry, 9.9% of patients developed cardiogenic shock, 17.3% of patients required invasive or noninvasive ventilation, and 8.6% of patients had cardiopulmonary resuscitation.[13] The incidence of cardiac arrest among hospitalized patients with SIC was approximately 5%.[14] Independent predictors of acute heart failure include advanced age, low LVEF at presentation, higher admission and peak troponin levels, and a physical stressor preceding the onset of symptoms.[2,53]

At least 3 different patterns of regional LV wall motion abnormalities have been identified in patients with SIC, classified as apical ballooning (**Figs. 1** and **2**), midventricular ballooning, and basal ballooning. Apical ballooning, being the most common pattern, occurs in 70% to 80% of cases. The midventricular ballooning pattern and basal ballooning occur in about 10% to 20% and 1% to 2% of patients with SIC, respectively. Other variant morphologies, such as inverted, right ventricular involvement, or focal forms, have also been described.[2,3,54] Sex differences in the morphologies of ventricular dysfunction have not been reported. Myocardial hypokinesis or akinesis is usually circumferential beyond the territory of a single coronary artery distribution. This unique feature of SIC is helpful for differentiating from ACS. Aside from hypokinetic segments, the rest of the myocardium is usually hyperkinetic to compensate for decreased LVEF and cardiac output. LV wall motion abnormalities are often completely reversible, which is a diagnostic character of SIC.

Left ventricular overflow tract obstruction LV outflow tract (LVOT) obstruction occurs to 10% to 25% of patients with SIC.[2,3,55] LVOT obstruction (**Fig. 3**), often accompanied by mitral regurgitation, is a result of hypercontraction of the basal LV myocardium, systolic anterior motion of the mitral

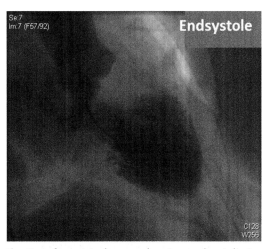

Fig. 2. Left ventriculogram showing end-systolic image of an apical ballooning morphology.

valve, or apical subvalvular tethering. It is more common with the apical ballooning pattern and it may be provoked or exacerbated by catecholamine drugs used to treat hypotension. In 32 patients with SIC, 6 patients were diagnosed with significant LVOT obstruction. Older age, septal bulging, systolic anterior motion, mitral regurgitation, and hemodynamic instability were associated with this condition.[55] In a series of 136 patients with SIC, 13 patients developed dynamic obstruction to LVOT (gradients of 54 ± 48 mm Hg); it developed in 7 patients after intravenous administration of inotropic agents for hypotension.[14] In 227 patients with SIC enrolled in the Takotsubo Italian Network, LVOT obstruction was found to be more prevalent in patients with major adverse events (23.7%) compared with patients without adverse events (8.9%).[56] In the German registry, an LV pressure gradient (20–100 mm Hg) was

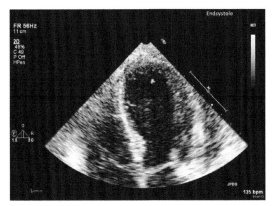

Fig. 1. Echocardiogram showing end-systolic image of an apical ballooning morphology.

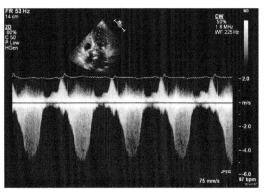

Fig. 3. Continuous wave Doppler interrogation showing left ventricular outflow tract obstruction with peak gradient of 95 mm Hg.

documented in 10 of 209 patients with SIC. In the patient with the highest gradient, epinephrine had been administered because of cardiogenic shock and LVOT gradient rapidly resolved after discontinuation of the catecholamine infusion.[53]

Arrhythmia Arrhythmia is common in patients with SIC. New atrial fibrillation has been reported in 5% to 15% of cases and ventricular arrhythmia occurs in 4% to 10% of patients during the acute phase. Potentially lethal arrhythmia, including ventricular fibrillation, torsades de pointes, and ventricular tachycardia, can occur at presentation or during hospitalization in less than 5% of patients.[2,3,57] Ventricular tachycardia and sudden cardiac arrest occurred significantly more often in males than in females. Atrial fibrillation was significantly less in males compared with females. Independent predictors of ventricular arrhythmia were syncope, atypical pattern of SIC, high troponin peak, dobutamine use, and relatively young age in the female and menopausal population. During follow-up, no significant difference in mortality rate was found between patients with or without ventricular arrhythmia.[11] In a series of 93 patients with SIC, 8.6% of patients experienced ventricular fibrillation or torsades de pointes, in which 6 patients had pause-dependent torsades de pointes or ventricular fibrillation in the setting of substantial QT prolongation.[58] The National Inpatient Sample database found atrial fibrillation in 6.9%, ventricular tachycardia in 3.2%, and ventricular fibrillation or ventricular flutter in 1% of patients with SIC.

Embolic events Ventricular thrombi are reported in 2.5% to 8.0% of patients with SIC, and can lead to systemic or pulmonary embolic events (**Fig. 4**).[2,3,59] It can occur either at initial presentation or at any time later during the disease course. LV wall motion abnormalities and decreased LVEF were thought to be the causes; however, recent studies suggested coagulation cascade might contribute to thromboemboli in patients with SIC.[60] Patients should be treated with a longer course (usually 3 months) of therapeutic anticoagulation and follow-up imaging is helpful to monitor resolution of ventricular thrombi. In 541 patients with SIC enrolled in the German Italian Stress Cardiomyopathy Registry, 12 patients (2.2%) developed LV thrombi and these patients were all female presenting with an apical ballooning pattern. These patients were all treated with oral anticoagulation therapy; however, 2 patients suffered a cerebrovascular accident before treatment initiation. A high troponin level (>10 ng/mL) was an independent predictor of LV thrombi. At long-term follow-up, the survival rate is not

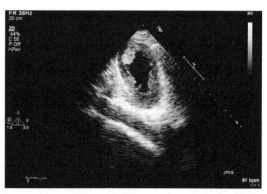

Fig. 4. Echocardiogram showing a thrombus located at the apex of the left ventricle.

different between patients with or without LV thrombi.[61]

Role of biomarkers The majority of patients with SIC (>90%) had mild troponin and creatine kinase elevation. The increase in cardiac enzymes is disproportionally low to the extent of LV wall motion abnormalities and LV dysfunction in comparison with ACS.[2,3] B-type natriuretic peptide (BNP) and N-terminal pro-BNP (NT-proBNP) are valuable markers of myocardial deterioration and recovery. During the acute phase of SIC, serum BNP or NT-proBNP are almost universally elevated and their levels do not correlate with cardiac hemodynamic indices. The magnitude of BNP elevation is higher in SIC compared with in ACS.[62]

Studies also suggested high NT-proBNP/myoglobin, NT-proBNP/troponin T, and BNP/creatine kinase-MB ratios can be instrumental for the differential diagnosis of ACS and SIC.[63] BNP levels and BNP/troponin I ratio were significantly higher in SIC compared with those in ST-elevation myocardial infarction and non–ST-elevation myocardial infarction.[64] SIC can be distinguished from ACS with a 95% specificity with the use of the BNP/troponin T ratio of 1272 or greater (sensitivity of 52%) and a BNP/creatine kinase-MB ratio of 29.9 or greater (sensitivity of 50%).[65] Elevated serum catecholamines (epinephrine, norepinephrine, and dopamine), neuropeptide-Y, and serotonin levels were also reported in patients with SIC.

Role of imaging Transthoracic echocardiography is the first-line noninvasive imaging modality for the evaluation of patients with suspected SIC. Transthoracic echocardiography, together with hemodynamic assessment with color Doppler interrogation, can be obtained quickly at the acute phase of presentation to assess LV dysfunction (see **Fig. 1**) and to detect potential complications, such as LVOT obstruction (see **Fig. 3**), ventricular thrombi (see **Fig. 4**), mitral regurgitation, right ventricular involvement, and cardiac rupture, among others. Such information is key to successful management of these patients, as well as risk stratification and monitoring recovery.[66] Myocardial contrast echocardiography can be used to assess coronary microcirculation integrity and perfusion defects in the acute phase of SIC. Myocardial contrast echocardiography is also useful to monitor the gradual improvement of microcirculatory function during recovery phase, which usually occurs before the recovery of LVEF and regional wall motion abnormalities.[21,67] Global longitudinal strain by speckle tracking echocardiography is a sensitive technique for the assessment of myocardial deformation before apparent LV dysfunction and wall motion abnormalities occur.[68,69]

CMR has emerged over the past decade as an important noninvasive imaging tool for the diagnosis and follow-up of patients with SIC because of its unique ability to obtain myocardial tissue characterization. The presence of diffuse or transmural distribution of edema on T2-weighted CMR and the absence of LGE are key features to distinguish from ACS. In 59 patients who presented with ACS and an apical ballooning pattern on left ventriculography, but normal coronary arteries, CMR revealed 13 patients (22%) with a diagnosis of myocardial infarction, 8 patients (13.6%) with a diagnosis of myocarditis, and 38 patients (64.4%) with suspected SIC.[70] This study suggests that CMR can be instrumental in differentiating SIC from myocarditis and coronary emboli with spontaneous lysis.

Single-photon emission computed tomography (SPECT) and PET can be good supplemental modalities in SIC to assess myocardial innervation, metabolism and coronary flow.[54] ^{123}I-meta-iodobenzylguanidine imaging offers the unique possibility of investigating cardiac sympathetic innervation. Impairment of myocardial blood flow and coronary flow reserve assessed by PET unproportional to epicardial CAD indicates microvascular dysfunction. Studies with PET also showed reduced glucose or fatty acid metabolism in myocardium and the extent of metabolic defect was found to be more severe than perfusion abnormality.[24–27]

Treatment

Supportive measures are the mainstay of management of SIC to sustain life and to minimize complications.[2,71] There are no randomized clinical trials to support specific treatment of SIC. Patients generally are treated with aspirin, beta-blockers, angiotensin-converting enzyme inhibitors (ACEi)/angiotensin receptor blockers (ARB) owing to LV dysfunction, and intravenous diuretics if needed

for volume overload and pulmonary edema. Data regarding these treatments are mostly from small retrospective studies and there is no proven benefit in improving outcomes.[72]

Beta-blocker therapy was thought to be beneficial owing to its suppression of excessive catecholamine stimulation in SIC. Beta-blockers can be also considered in patients with atrial or ventricular tachyarrhythmias when they are hemodynamically stable. However, a large retrospective cohort from Japan (2672 patients) revealed no significant difference in 30-day in-hospital mortality between patients who started beta-blockers on hospitalization day 1 or 2 and those who did not receive beta-blockers during hospitalization.[73] Similarly, there was no survival benefit of using beta-blockers at 1 year in the International Takotsubo Registry.[13]

Studies showed that patients with SIC may have low peripheral vascular resistance owing to altered peripheral sympathetic nerve activity, so vasoactive drugs, such as ACEi, need to be used with caution, especially in the acute phase. However, the use of ACEi/ARB was associated with improved survival at 1 year.[13] Metaanalyses also suggested the tendency of reducing the risk of recurrence with ACEi/ARB.[74,75] In the absence of data from randomized clinical trials, the appropriate duration of any therapy is unclear.

Hypotension in the setting of LVOT obstruction may warrant stopping epinephrine or nonepinephirne and administering beta-blockers and phenylephrine.[76] In severe cases complicated by progressive circulatory failure and cardiogenic shock, catecholamine-sparing positive inotropic agents, or early mechanical support, such as intra-aortic balloon pump or extracorporeal membrane oxygenation, should be considered. Cases of SIC successfully treated with milrinone have been reported,[77,78] but dobutamine should be avoided because it can precipitate or worsen catecholamine-induced myocardial stunning and LVOT obstruction.

The evidence of long-term follow-up of SIC is lacking. Patients with SIC should be followed for at least 3 to 6 months after discharge. The follow-up should include history, physical examination, review of medications, ECG, and imaging to assess recovery of LV function and regional wall motion abnormalities.[2] For patients with a history of ventricular thrombi, the resolution of the thrombi should be confirmed before withdrawing anticoagulation.

Prognosis

The most characteristic hallmark of SIC is reversible LV dysfunction; thus, the prognosis of SIC was thought to be benign. The recovery process usually takes 1 to 2 weeks, but can vary between a few hours to longer than 2 months. However, increasing evidence suggests a high incidence of complications and substantial mortality and recurrence. The mortality associated with SIC is similar to that of ACS,[79] with the in-hospital mortality being 2% to 5% and the 5-year mortality being 3% to 17%.[2] According to the National Inpatient Sample database, in-hospital mortality was 4.2%. The mean duration of stay was 6.1 ± 15.9 days. Neither age nor race was associated with mortality. Male gender was associated with higher in-hospital mortality.[13,47,48] The International Takotsubo Registry revealed that patients with SIC and ACS had similar rates of severe inpatient complications and independent predictors of these complications included physical triggers, acute neurologic/psychiatric diseases, elevated troponin levels, and low LVEF.[13] During long-term follow-up, the rate of major adverse cardiac and cerebrovascular events was 9.9% per patient-year and the rate of death was 5.6% per patient-year.[13] A recent metaanalysis including 37 studies (2120 patients with SIC) showed the in-hospital mortality rate of SIC was 4.5% (range, 3.1%–6.2%). Among all deaths, 38% were directly related to complications and the rest to underlying noncardiac conditions. Male gender was associated with a higher mortality rate.[74]

Research on the long-term outcomes of SIC is limited. In a case-control study with 37 patients recovered from prior SIC more than 12 months before enrollment, 88% of patients with a history of SIC demonstrated persisting symptoms compatible with heart failure and cardiac limitation on exercise testing. Despite normal LVEF and serum biomarkers after recovery, persistent long-term myocardial impairment was demonstrated by reduced cardiac deformation indices on speckle tracking echocardiography, increased native T1 mapping values on CMR, and impaired cardiac energetic status.[80]

SIC may recur in 5% to 22% of cases.[2,3] A recent metaanalysis based on 31 cohorts indicated that the cumulative incidence of recurrence was approximately 5% at 6 years and the annual rate of recurrence was approximately 1% to 2%.[74] Nearly all cases of recurrence occurred in women. The recurrence rate was inversely correlated with ACEi/ARB prescription, but not with beta-blocker prescription.[74] The International Takotsubo Registry reported that the rate of recurrence was 1.8% per patient-year, with a span of 25 days up to 9.2 years after the first event.[13]

SUMMARY

SIC is characterized by reversible myocardial injury with distinctive regional wall motion abnormalities usually precipitated by a significant emotional or physical stressor. This condition has a strong predilection for older women and has a trend of increasing incidence in the recent decades. The diagnosis and differential diagnosis of SIC can be challenging. Supportive measures are the mainstay of management. The prognosis of this condition is not benign owing to substantial morbidity and mortality. Current evidence of management is mostly from small retrospective studies and larger randomized prospective studies are warranted to investigate treatment options.

REFERENCES

1. Schneider B, Athanasiadis A, Stollberger C, et al. Gender differences in the manifestation of takotsubo cardiomyopathy. Int J Cardiol 2013;166(3): 584–8.
2. Lyon AR, Bossone E, Schneider B, et al. Current state of knowledge on Takotsubo syndrome: a Position Statement from the Taskforce on Takotsubo Syndrome of the Heart Failure Association of the European Society of Cardiology. Eur J Heart Fail 2016;18(1):8–27.
3. Sharkey SW. A clinical perspective of the Takotsubo Syndrome. Heart Fail Clin 2016;12(4):507–20.
4. Dote K, Sato H, Tateishi H, et al. Myocardial stunning due to simultaneous multivessel coronary spasms: a review of 5 cases. J Cardiol 1991;21(2):203–14 [in Japanese].
5. Deshmukh A, Kumar G, Pant S, et al. Prevalence of Takotsubo cardiomyopathy in the United States. Am Heart J 2012;164(1):66–71.e61.
6. Bertoni AG, Bonds DE, Thom T, et al. Acute coronary syndrome national statistics: challenges in definitions. Am Heart J 2005;149(6):1055–61.
7. Minhas AS, Hughey AB, Kolias TJ. Nationwide trends in reported incidence of Takotsubo Cardiomyopathy from 2006 to 2012. Am J Cardiol 2015; 116(7):1128–31.
8. Eshtehardi P, Koestner SC, Adorjan P, et al. Transient apical ballooning syndrome–clinical characteristics, ballooning pattern, and long-term follow-up in a Swiss population. Int J Cardiol 2009;135(3):370–5.
9. Previtali M, Repetto A, Panigada S, et al. Left ventricular apical ballooning syndrome: prevalence, clinical characteristics and pathogenetic mechanisms in a European population. Int J Cardiol 2009;134(1):91–6.
10. Kurowski V, Kaiser A, von Hof K, et al. Apical and midventricular transient left ventricular dysfunction syndrome (tako-tsubo cardiomyopathy): frequency,

mechanisms, and prognosis. Chest 2007;132(3): 809–16.

11. Auzel O, Mustafic H, Pilliere R, et al. Incidence, characteristics, risk factors, and outcomes of Takotsubo Cardiomyopathy with and without ventricular arrhythmia. Am J Cardiol 2016;117(8):1242–7.

12. Donohue D, Movahed MR. Clinical characteristics, demographics and prognosis of transient left ventricular apical ballooning syndrome. Heart Fail Rev 2005;10(4):311–6.

13. Templin C, Ghadri JR, Diekmann J, et al. Clinical features and outcomes of Takotsubo (stress) cardiomyopathy. N Engl J Med 2015;373(10):929–38.

14. Sharkey SW, Windenburg DC, Lesser JR, et al. Natural history and expansive clinical profile of stress (tako-tsubo) cardiomyopathy. J Am Coll Cardiol 2010;55(4):333–41.

15. Schneider B, Sechtem U. Influence of age and gender in Takotsubo syndrome. Heart Fail Clin 2016;12(4):521–30.

16. Lindsay J, Paixao A, Chao T, et al. Pathogenesis of the Takotsubo syndrome: a unifying hypothesis. Am J Cardiol 2010;106(9):1360–3.

17. Pelliccia F, Kaski JC, Crea F, et al. Pathophysiology of Takotsubo syndrome. Circulation 2017;135(24): 2426–41.

18. Akashi YJ, Nef HM, Lyon AR. Epidemiology and pathophysiology of Takotsubo syndrome. Nat Rev Cardiol 2015;12(7):387–97.

19. Nazir S, Lohani S, Tachamo N, et al. Takotsubo cardiomyopathy associated with epinephrine use: a systematic review and meta-analysis. Int J Cardiol 2017;229:67–70.

20. Vitale C, Rosano GM, Kaski JC. Role of coronary microvascular dysfunction in Takotsubo cardiomyopathy. Circ J 2016;80(2):299–305.

21. Abdelmoneim SS, Mankad SV, Bernier M, et al. Microvascular function in Takotsubo cardiomyopathy with contrast echocardiography: prospective evaluation and review of literature. J Am Soc Echocardiogr 2009;22(11):1249–55.

22. Khalid N, Iqbal I, Coram R, et al. Thrombolysis in myocardial infarction frame count in Takotsubo cardiomyopathy. Int J Cardiol 2015;191:107–8.

23. Galiuto L, De Caterina AR, Porfidia A, et al. Reversible coronary microvascular dysfunction: a common pathogenetic mechanism in Apical Ballooning or Tako-Tsubo Syndrome. Eur Heart J 2010;31(11): 1319–27.

24. Cimarelli S, Sauer F, Morel O, et al. Transient left ventricular dysfunction syndrome: patho-physiological bases through nuclear medicine imaging. Int J Cardiol 2010;144(2):212–8.

25. Matsuo S, Nakajima K, Kinuya S, et al. Diagnostic utility of 123I-BMIPP imaging in patients with Takotsubo cardiomyopathy. J Cardiol 2014;64(1): 49–56.

26. Owa M, Aizawa K, Urasawa N, et al. Emotional stress-induced 'ampulla cardiomyopathy': discrepancy between the metabolic and sympathetic innervation imaging performed during the recovery course. Jpn Circ J 2001;65(4):349–52.

27. Christensen TE, Bang LE, Holmvang L, et al. Cardiac (9)(9)mTc sestamibi SPECT and (1)(8)F FDG PET as viability markers in Takotsubo cardiomyopathy. Int J Cardiovasc Imaging 2014;30(7):1407–16.

28. Gaibazzi N, Ugo F, Vignali L, et al. Tako-Tsubo cardiomyopathy with coronary artery stenosis: a case-series challenging the original definition. Int J Cardiol 2009;133(2):205–12.

29. Kurisu S, Inoue I, Kawagoe T, et al. Prevalence of incidental coronary artery disease in tako-tsubo cardiomyopathy. Coron Artery Dis 2009;20(3):214–8.

30. Ibanez B, Benezet-Mazuecos J, Navarro F, et al. Takotsubo syndrome: a Bayesian approach to interpreting its pathogenesis. Mayo Clin Proc 2006; 81(6):732–5.

31. Eitel I, Stiermaier T, Graf T, et al. Optical coherence tomography to evaluate plaque burden and morphology in patients with Takotsubo syndrome. J Am Heart Assoc 2016;5(12) [pii:e004474].

32. Prasad A, Lerman A, Rihal CS. Apical ballooning syndrome (Tako-Tsubo or stress cardiomyopathy): a mimic of acute myocardial infarction. Am Heart J 2008;155(3):408–17.

33. Kawai S, Kitabatake A, Tomoike H. Guidelines for diagnosis of Takotsubo (ampulla) cardiomyopathy. Circ J 2007;71(6):990–2.

34. Parodi G, Citro R, Bellandi B, et al. Revised clinical diagnostic criteria for Tako-tsubo syndrome: the Tako-tsubo Italian Network proposal. Int J Cardiol 2014;172(1):282–3.

35. Eitel I, von Knobelsdorff-Brenkenhoff F, Bernhardt P, et al. Clinical characteristics and cardiovascular magnetic resonance findings in stress (Takotsubo) cardiomyopathy. Jama 2011;306(3):277–86.

36. Scantlebury DC, Prasad A. Diagnosis of Takotsubo cardiomyopathy. Circ J 2014;78(9):2129–39.

37. Madias JE. Why the current diagnostic criteria of Takotsubo syndrome are outmoded: a proposal for new criteria. Int J Cardiol 2014;174(3):468–70.

38. Lee SR, Lee SE, Rhee TM, et al. Discrimination of stress (Takotsubo) cardiomyopathy from acute coronary syndrome with clinical risk factors and coronary evaluation in real-world clinical practice. Int J Cardiol 2017;235:154–61.

39. Zorzi A, Baritussio A, ElMaghawry M, et al. Differential diagnosis at admission between Takotsubo cardiomyopathy and acute apical-anterior myocardial infarction in postmenopausal women. Eur Heart J Acute Cardiovasc Care 2016;5(4):298–307.

40. Cortadellas J, Figueras J, Llibre C, et al. Acute cardiac syndromes without significant coronary stenosis: differential features between myocardial infarction

and apical-ballooning syndrome. Coron Artery Dis 2011;22(6):435–41.

41. Tamura A, Watanabe T, Ishihara M, et al. A new electrocardiographic criterion to differentiate between Takotsubo cardiomyopathy and anterior wall ST-segment elevation acute myocardial infarction. Am J Cardiol 2011;108(5):630–3.

42. Kosuge M, Kimura K. Electrocardiographic findings of Takotsubo cardiomyopathy as compared with those of anterior acute myocardial infarction. J Electrocardiol 2014;47(5):684–9.

43. Frangieh AH, Obeid S, Ghadri JR, et al. ECG criteria to differentiate between Takotsubo (stress) cardiomyopathy and myocardial infarction. J Am Heart Assoc 2016;5(6) [pii:e003418].

44. Jaguszewski M, Osipova J, Ghadri JR, et al. A signature of circulating microRNAs differentiates Takotsubo cardiomyopathy from acute myocardial infarction. Eur Heart J 2014;35(15):999–1006.

45. Caforio AL, Tona F, Vinci A, et al. Acute biopsy-proven lymphocytic myocarditis mimicking Takotsubo cardiomyopathy. Eur J Heart Fail 2009;11(4):428–31.

46. Murakami T, Yoshikawa T, Maekawa Y, et al. Gender differences in patients with Takotsubo cardiomyopathy: multi-center registry from Tokyo CCU Network. PLoS One 2015;10(8):e0136655.

47. Brinjikji W, El-Sayed AM, Salka S. In-hospital mortality among patients with Takotsubo cardiomyopathy: a study of the National Inpatient Sample 2008 to 2009. Am Heart J 2012;164(2):215–21.

48. Weidner KJ, El-Battrawy I, Behnes M, et al. Sex differences of in-hospital outcome and long-term mortality in patients with Takotsubo cardiomyopathy. Ther Clin Risk Manag 2017;13:863–9.

49. Dias A, Franco E, Koshkelashvili N, et al. Racial and ethnic differences in Takotsubo cardiomyopathy presentation and outcomes. Int J Cardiol 2015;194:100–3.

50. Kao DP, Kreso E. Gender and racial differences in demographics and outcomes in 800 inpatient admissions for Takotsubo cardiomyopathy [abstract]. J Am Coll Cardiol 2011;57(14). supplement, E264.

51. Franco E, Dias A, Koshkelashvili N, et al. Distinctive electrocardiographic features in African Americans diagnosed with Takotsubo Cardiomyopathy. Ann Noninvasive Electrocardiol 2016;21(5):486–92.

52. Madhavan M, Rihal CS, Lerman A, et al. Acute heart failure in apical ballooning syndrome (TakoTsubo/stress cardiomyopathy): clinical correlates and Mayo Clinic risk score. J Am Coll Cardiol 2011;57(12):1400–1.

53. Schneider B, Athanasiadis A, Schwab J, et al. Complications in the clinical course of tako-tsubo cardiomyopathy. Int J Cardiol 2014;176(1):199–205.

54. Citro R, Pontone G, Pace L, et al. Contemporary imaging in Takotsubo syndrome. Heart Fail Clin 2016;12(4):559–75.

55. De Backer O, Debonnaire P, Gevaert S, et al. Prevalence, associated factors and management implications of left ventricular outflow tract obstruction in Takotsubo cardiomyopathy: a two-year, two-center experience. BMC Cardiovasc Disord 2014;14:147.

56. Citro R, Rigo F, D'Andrea A, et al. Echocardiographic correlates of acute heart failure, cardiogenic shock, and in-hospital mortality in tako-tsubo cardiomyopathy. JACC Cardiovasc Imaging 2014;7(2):119–29.

57. Syed FF, Asirvatham SJ, Francis J. Arrhythmia occurrence with Takotsubo cardiomyopathy: a literature review. Europace 2011;13(6):780–8.

58. Madias C, Fitzgibbons TP, Alsheikh-Ali AA, et al. Acquired long QT syndrome from stress cardiomyopathy is associated with ventricular arrhythmias and torsades de pointes. Heart Rhythm 2011;8(4):555–61.

59. El-Battrawy I, Borggrefe M, Akin I. Takotsubo syndrome and embolic events. Heart Fail Clin 2016;12(4):543–50.

60. Cecchi E, Parodi G, Fatucchi S, et al. Prevalence of thrombophilic disorders in Takotsubo patients: the (ThROmbophylia in TAkotsubo cardiomyopathy) TROTA study. Clin Res Cardiol 2016;105(9):717–26.

61. Santoro F, Stiermaier T, Tarantino N, et al. Left ventricular thrombi in Takotsubo syndrome: incidence, predictors, and management: results from the GEIST (German Italian Stress Cardiomyopathy) Registry. J Am Heart Assoc 2017;6(12) [pii:e006990].

62. Ahmed KA, Madhavan M, Prasad A. Brain natriuretic peptide in apical ballooning syndrome (Takotsubo/stress cardiomyopathy): comparison with acute myocardial infarction. Coron Artery Dis 2012;23(4):259–64.

63. Frohlich GM, Schoch B, Schmid F, et al. Takotsubo cardiomyopathy has a unique cardiac biomarker profile: NT-proBNP/myoglobin and NT-proBNP/troponin T ratios for the differential diagnosis of acute coronary syndromes and stress induced cardiomyopathy. Int J Cardiol 2012;154(3):328–32.

64. Doyen D, Moceri P, Chiche O, et al. Cardiac biomarkers in Takotsubo cardiomyopathy. Int J Cardiol 2014;174(3):798–801.

65. Randhawa MS, Dhillon AS, Taylor HC, et al. Diagnostic utility of cardiac biomarkers in discriminating Takotsubo cardiomyopathy from acute myocardial infarction. J Card Fail 2014;20(5):377.e25-31.

66. Citro R, Lyon AR, Meimoun P, et al. Standard and advanced echocardiography in Takotsubo (stress) cardiomyopathy: clinical and prognostic implications. J Am Soc Echocardiogr 2015;28(1):57–74.

67. Jain M, Upadaya S, Zarich SW. Serial evaluation of microcirculatory dysfunction in patients with Takotsubo cardiomyopathy by myocardial contrast echocardiography. Clin Cardiol 2013;36(9):531–4.

68. Heggemann F, Hamm K, Kaelsch T, et al. Global and regional myocardial function quantification in Takotsubo cardiomyopathy in comparison to acute anterior myocardial infarction using two-dimensional (2D) strain echocardiography. Echocardiography 2011;28(7):715–9.

69. Sosa S, Banchs J. Early recognition of apical ballooning syndrome by global longitudinal strain using speckle tracking imaging–the evil eye pattern, a case series. Echocardiography 2015;32(7): 1184–92.

70. Eitel I, Behrendt F, Schindler K, et al. Differential diagnosis of suspected apical ballooning syndrome using contrast-enhanced magnetic resonance imaging. Eur Heart J 2008;29(21):2651–9.

71. Omerovic E. Takotsubo syndrome-scientific basis for current treatment strategies. Heart Fail Clin 2016; 12(4):577–86.

72. Santoro F, Ieva R, Musaico F, et al. Lack of efficacy of drug therapy in preventing Takotsubo cardiomyopathy recurrence: a meta-analysis. Clin Cardiol 2014;37(7):434–9.

73. Isogai T, Matsui H, Tanaka H, et al. Early β-blocker use and in-hospital mortality in patients with Takotsubo cardiomyopathy. Heart 2016;102(13): 1029–35.

74. Singh K, Carson K, Usmani Z, et al. Systematic review and meta-analysis of incidence and correlates of recurrence of Takotsubo cardiomyopathy. Int J Cardiol 2014;174(3):696–701.

75. Brunetti ND, Santoro F, De Gennaro L, et al. Drug treatment rates with beta-blockers and ACE-inhibitors/angiotensin receptor blockers and recurrences in Takotsubo cardiomyopathy: a meta-regression analysis. Int J Cardiol 2016;214:340–2.

76. Angue M, Soubirou L, Vandroux D, et al. Beneficial effects of intravenous beta-blockers in Tako-Tsubo syndrome with dynamic left ventricular outflow tract obstruction and severe haemodynamic impairment. Int J Cardiol 2014;177(2):e56–7.

77. Mrozek S, Srairi M, Marhar F, et al. Successful treatment of inverted Takotsubo cardiomyopathy after severe traumatic brain injury with milrinone after dobutamine failure. Heart Lung 2016;45(5):406–8.

78. Doyen D, Dellamonica J, Moceri P, et al. Tako-Tsubo cardiomyopathy presenting with cardiogenic shock successfully treated with milrinone: a case report. Heart Lung 2014;43(4):331–3.

79. Redfors B, Vedad R, Angeras O, et al. Mortality in Takotsubo syndrome is similar to mortality in myocardial infarction - A report from the SWEDEHEART registry. Int J Cardiol 2015;185:282–9.

80. Scally C, Rudd A, Mezincescu A, et al. Persistent long-term structural, functional, and metabolic changes after stress-induced (Takotsubo) cardiomyopathy. Circulation 2018;137(10):1039–48.

Atrial Fibrillation and Heart Failure in Women

Nidhi Madan, MD, MPH[a], Dipti Itchhaporia, MD[b], Christine M. Albert, MD, MPH[c], Neelum T. Aggarwal, MD[d], Annabelle Santos Volgman, MD[e],*

KEYWORDS

- Women • Rate control • Rhythm control • Systolic heart failure
- Diastolic heart failure atrial fibrillation

KEY POINTS

- Women with atrial fibrillation have a higher incidence of heart failure with preserved ejection fraction compared with men.
- Women who have heart failure with preserved ejection fraction are at a higher risk of atrial fibrillation, hospitalizations, and all adverse cardiovascular events than men.
- Women with atrial fibrillation have a higher risk of stroke than men when treated with warfarin but not when treated with novel anticoagulants, yet women are significantly undertreated with them.
- Women are treated with digoxin more often than men, despite evidence of increased mortality and increased risk of breast cancer with its use.
- Women have higher procedural risks from catheter ablation, and they are not well-represented in ablation studies.

INTRODUCTION

Atrial fibrillation (AF) and heart failure (HF) have emerged as 2 new epidemics of cardiovascular disease, with hospitalizations doubling for each diagnosis since 1984.[1] A recent study based on the Framingham Heart Study cohort showed that men have a higher lifetime risk of developing AF compared with women.[2] However, women with AF have a greater risk of strokes and increased mortality compared with men.[3] Combined, AF and HF cause substantial morbidity, mortality, and health care costs, and both contribute to the incidence of stroke and cognitive decline in women. In individuals with AF, deaths caused by HF (30%) exceeded deaths caused by stroke (8%).[4] Excellent reviews have been published on AF and HF.[5,6] This review examines factors contributing to the poorer outcomes seen in women with AF and HF compared with those seen in men. A further understanding of the mechanisms and predisposing factors underlying the evolving epidemics of HF and AF is needed to establish optimal treatment and prevention strategies. Such strategies will likely vary for women compared with men, given the important sex differences that exist in AF and HF incidence, risk factors, and outcomes.

Disclosure: C.M. Albert receives NIH grants. The other authors have nothing to disclose.
[a] Department of Medicine, Cardiology Division, Rush University Medical Center, 1653 West Congress Parkway, Chicago, IL 60612, USA; [b] Department of Medicine, Cardiology Division, Hoag Memorial Hospital, University of California, Irvine, 520 Superior Avenue, Newport Beach, CA 92663, USA; [c] Department of Medicine, Cardiology Division, Brigham and Women's Medical Center, 75 Francis Street Towers 3a, Boston, MA 02115, USA; [d] Department of Neurological Sciences, Rush Alzheimer's Disease Center, Rush University Medical Center, 1750 W. Harrison, Suite 1000, Chicago, IL 60612, USA; [e] Department of Medicine, Cardiology Division, Rush University Medical Center, 1725 W. Harrison Street, Room 1159, Chicago, IL 60612, USA
* Corresponding author.
E-mail address: Annabelle_Volgman@rush.edu

POORER OUTCOMES IN WOMEN WITH ATRIAL FIBRILLATION AND HEART FAILURE COMPARED WITH THOSE SEEN IN MEN

Often coexisting with HF, AF and is both a risk factor for and consequence of HF with preserved ejection fraction (HFpEF; 55%–65%) and HF with reduced ejection fraction (HFrEF; ≤40%).[7] The coexistence of AF and HF may result in poor cardiovascular outcomes.[8,9] Preexisting AF was associated with a greater 3-year risk of all-cause mortality and hospital readmissions for stroke, HF, and AF in both men and women.[10] A metaanalysis of 30 cohort studies showed that AF is associated with a higher relative risk of cardiovascular and all-cause mortality, stroke, and HF in women compared with men.[11] In AF participants in the Framingham Heart Study, the development of HF was associated with rates of mortality almost three times higher in both men and women. However, in HF subjects, the development of AF was associated with a 60% increase in mortality in men but a 170% increase in mortality in women.[9]

In the Women's Health Study, of the 34,000 postmenopausal women who did not have prevalent cardiovascular disease at baseline, 1495 developed AF after a median follow-up of 20.6 years. Women with new-onset AF without prevalent HF had a significantly increased (9-fold) risk of developing HF. When women with existing AF developed HF, they had a significant increase in all-cause mortality (hazard ratio, 1.83; 95% confidence interval [CI], 1.37–2.45) and cardiovascular mortality (hazard ratio, 2.87; 95% CI, 1.70–4.85).[12] Modifiable risk factors, including smoking, obesity, hypertension, and diabetes, accounted for the majority of population attributable risk of HF in women with AF. Thus, modification of risk factors may lower HF risk in women with AF.

ELECTRICAL AND STRUCTURAL CHANGES IN THE ATRIA OF PATIENTS WITH HEART FAILURE

Patients with AF or HF have several risk factors in common (**Fig. 1**). These multiple risk factors may cause changes in the structural and electrical properties of the heart and may have different effects in men compared with women. Women have physiologically smaller hearts, more coronary microvascular dysfunction, higher resting left ventricular ejection fraction, and longer baseline repolarization corrected QT intervals.[13–15]

Patients with HFpEF have left atrial enlargement, decreased left atrial function, and increased left atrial stiffness compared with controls.[16] Patients with a severely decreased left ventricular ejection fraction have atrial remodeling and higher AF inducibility.[17] Both types of HF cause an upregulation of the renin–angiotensin–aldosterone system axis that is, implicated in the development of cardiac fibrosis.[18]

SEX DIFFERENCES IN ATRIAL FIBRILLATION AND HEART FAILURE

Epidemiologic studies show that the lifetime risk of developing HFpEF was similar in men and women, albeit slightly higher for women. However, compared with women, men had a higher risk of developing HF with a reduced ejection fraction of less than 40% (**Table 1**).[19] This was seen in the Framingham Heart Study, in which men had a higher cumulative incidence of HFrEF, but women had a similar incidence of HFpEF and HFrEF.[20]

In clinical studies, women have been found to develop HFpEF more often than men (**Fig. 2**).[21–23] Old age, hypertension, and sleep apnea are risk factors common to the development of both AF and HFpEF.[24] The risk of developing AF with HF is higher in women than men (in 1 study, the odds ratio was 5.9 for women and 4.5 for men).[25] Women with prevalent AF had a higher incidence of HFpEF compared with men (**Table 2**).[7]

CONGESTIVE HEART FAILURE AS A RISK FACTOR FOR STROKE IN ATRIAL FIBRILLATION

The $CHADS_2$ score, a stroke risk assessment for patients with AF, was introduced in 2001.[26] The $CHADS_2$ score assigns 1 point to each of 4 risk factors: congestive HF, hypertension, diabetes, and age 75 years or older, and 2 points to a history of stroke or transient ischemic attack. The CHA_2DS_2-VASC scale added female sex, age 65 to 74 years and vascular disease to the original $CHADS_2$, and it is now the recommended algorithm to determine the risk of stroke in patients with atrial fibrillation.[27] Each additional factor is given 1 point, with the exception of age 75 years or older, which is assigned 2 points. The CHA_2DS_2-VASC score designates 0 as low risk, 1 as moderate risk, and 2 or higher as high risk. Female sex and congestive HF both increase the risk of strokes in AF and are used as independent risk factors in the recommended stroke risk algorithm, CHA_2DS_2-VASC.[27] Whether HFrEF confers a higher risk of stroke than HFpEF in congestive HF patients was investigated in the PRESERVE study (Atrial Fibrillation and Outcomes in Heart Failure With Preserved vs Reduced Left Ventricular Ejection Fraction)[8] of 23,644 patients with a discharge diagnosis of congestive HF. In this

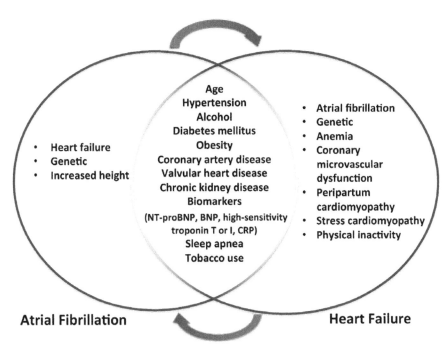

Fig. 1. Risk factors for the development of atrial fibrillation and heart failure in women. CRP, C-reactive protein. (*Data from* Refs.[12,68,69])

study, 48.3% of patients had documented AF (9081 preexisting, 2348 incident). Patients with preexisting AF and HFpEF had a higher risk of stroke than HFrEF patients. Furthermore, patients with incident AF and HFpEF had the highest risk of strokes compared with patients with HFrEF or patients with preexisting AF.[8]

The Treatment of Preserved Cardiac Function Heart Failure With an Aldosterone Antagonist Trial (TOPCAT) found that the association between incident AF and hospitalization was stronger in women than in men (63% vs 37%; $P_{interaction}$ = .032). In addition, in patients with AF, the risk

estimates for all adverse cardiovascular events (hospitalization for stroke, death, HF, and cardiovascular death) were higher in women than in men.[28] These studies have underscored the finding that women with diastolic dysfunction are vulnerable to the adverse effects of AF and HF.

ANTICOAGULATION AND STROKE PREVENTION IN ATRIAL FIBRILLATION AND HEART FAILURE

The substudy of Atrial Fibrillation Follow-up Investigation of Rhythm Management (AFFIRM) trial

Table 1
Lifetime risk for different HF phenotypes stratified by sex at selected index ages

Index Age (y)	Lifetime Risk, % (95% CI)					
	Overall HF		HFpEF		HFrEF	
	Women	Men	Women	Men	Women	Men
45	23.8 (22.4–25.1)	27.4 (25.9–29.0)	10.7 (9.6–11.8)	10.4 (9.1–11.6)	5.8 (5.03–6.6)	10.6 (9.4–11.8)
55	23.7 (22.4–25.0)	27.4 (25.9–29.0)	10.7 (9.6–11.8)	10.4 (9.2–11.6)	5.8 (5.0–6.6)	10.5 (9.3–11.8)
65	23.6 (22.3–25.0)	27.3 (25.8–28.9)	10.7 (9.5–11.8)	10.4 (9.1–11.6)	5.8 (5.0–6.6)	10.5 (9.2–11.7)
75	22.5 (21.1–23.8)	25.9 (24.3–27. 6)	10.3 (9.2–11.5)	9.7 (8.4–11.0)	5.2 (4.4–6.0)	9.5 (8.2–10.8)

Abbreviations: CI, confidence interval; HF, heart failure; HFpEF, heart failure with preserved ejection fraction; HFrEF, heart failure with reduced ejection fraction.

From Pandey A, Omar W, Ayers C, et al. Sex and race differences in lifetime risk of heart failure with preserved ejection fraction and heart failure with reduced ejection fraction. Circulation 2018;137(17):1816; with permission.

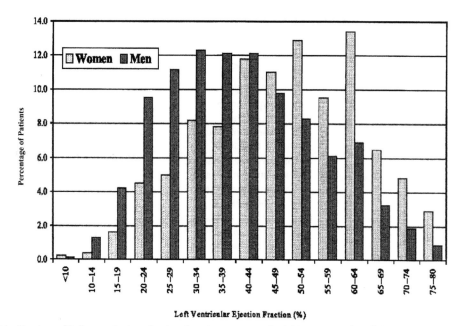

Fig. 2. Distribution of left ventricular ejection fraction measured within 12 months of the EuroHeart Failure survey among women (n = 2048; 41% of total enrolled) and men (n = 3249; 57% of total enrolled). When more than 1 ejection fraction measurement was available, the most recent one was used. Of those who did not drop out of the study, 51% of men but only 28% of women had a left ventricular ejection fraction of less than 40%. (*From* Hogg K, Swedberg K, McMurray J. Heart failure with preserved left ventricular systolic function; epidemiology, clinical characteristics, and prognosis. J Am Coll Cardiol 2004;43:323; with permission.)

showed that, in patients with AF, women had a higher risk of stroke compared with men, even with warfarin treatment. Women in the study spent more time outside or were below the therapeutic range. However, even in women who maintained a score within the therapeutic range ($\geq$66%), ischemic stroke rates were still higher compared with men (P = .009).[29] This sex disparity in the stroke risk of patients with AF was not seen with the use of novel anticoagulants. A metaanalysis evaluating sex differences in the residual risk of strokes and major bleeding in patients treated with warfarin compared with novel anticoagulants

showed similar stroke reduction in men and women when they were treated with novel anticoagulants.[30] Despite these results, women with AF were significantly less likely to receive oral anticoagulants than men at all levels of the CHA$_2$DS$_2$-VASC, as shown in the Practice INNovation And CLinical Excellence (PINNACLE) Registry (2008–2014).[31] The recommendation in the 2014 AF guidelines to use female sex as a risk factor may increase the use of anticoagulants in women.[27]

Another alternative to warfarin is percutaneous left atrial appendage closure, which is now available to prevent strokes in AF. In a 5-year outcome

Table 2
Sex-specific, age-standardized incidence rates of HF among those with AF

	Men	Women
	Incidence Rate per 1000 Person-Years (95% CI)	**Incidence Rate per 1000 Person-Years (95% CI)**
Incident HF	50.7 (41.9, 59.6)	56.0 (45.5, 66.6)
Incident HFpEF	21.2 (15.3, 27.0)	35.1 (26.9, 43.4)
Incident HFrEF	27.2 (20.8, 33.5)	12.4 (7.4, 17.4)

Abbreviations: AF, atrial fibrillation; CI, confidence interval; HF, heart failure; HFpEF, heart failure with preserved ejection fraction; HFrEF, heart failure with reduced ejection fraction.

From Santhanakrishnan R, Wang N, Larson MG, et al. Atrial fibrillation begets heart failure and vice versa: temporal associations and differences in preserved versus reduced ejection fraction. Circulation 2016;133:484–92; with permission.

analysis of left atrial appendage closure devices, the Watchman device was found to be noninferior to warfarin for the prevention of stroke, systemic embolism, and death, but the rate of adverse events was higher.[32] However, about 70% of study participants were male; therefore, the safety and efficacy of the Watchman device for women were not fully elucidated by this study.

RATE VERSUS RHYTHM CONTROL IN PATIENTS WITH ATRIAL FIBRILLATION AND HEART FAILURE

Theoretically, in patients with AF and HF, a rhythm control strategy should improve symptoms and survival. Patients with persistent AF who maintain sinus rhythm may experience an improvement in left ventricular function and a decrease in atrial size, although rate control has been shown to prevent the deterioration of left ventricular function.[33] Several studies have been conducted to determine whether rate versus rhythm control improved outcomes in patients with HF.

The AFFIRM and Rate Control versus Electrical Cardioversion (RACE) trials showed no difference in the outcomes of one strategy over the other.[34,35] Maintenance of sinus rhythm in patients with AF did not show survival benefits in clinical trials, which was most likely due to difficulty in achieving and maintaining sinus rhythm, especially in patients with HF. Difficulty in maintaining sinus rhythm was also seen in the study specifically in HF and AF, resulting in 21% of participants crossing over to the rate control arm from the rhythm control arm.[36] The trial also showed no difference in cardiovascular mortality between rate versus rhythm-control strategies in patients with HFrEF in the New York Heart Association functional classes II through IV.[36]

Despite experiencing more symptoms, women may be less likely to receive rhythm control treatment than men.[37] Sex-specific differences in the outcomes of rate versus rhythm control were evaluated in subgroup analyses of the AFFIRM and RACE trials. In the AFFIRM trial,[34] there was no sex-related difference in the risk of death between rate control and rhythm control strategies, although women were found to have a higher risk of stroke than men.[29] In the RACE study, although overall outcomes did not differ significantly by gender, women treated with rhythm control had a higher incidence of the primary endpoint (a composite of HF, pacemaker implantation, thromboembolic complications, cardiovascular mortality, and adverse effects of antiarrhythmic drugs) compared with age-matched women treated with rate control (32.0% vs 10.5%; absolute difference,

21.5%; 90% CI, 12.1%–30.8%). In men, the incidence of the primary endpoint did not differ significantly between the 2 treatment groups (17.2% vs 21.1%).[35] As a result of these studies, rate and rhythm strategies can be seen as acceptable treatments for patients with AF.

The presence of comorbid HF increases adverse outcomes. As discussed elsewhere in this article, women have poorer outcomes than men. The mechanisms contributing to this sex difference in each treatment strategy will now be discussed.

Rate Control Strategy

Atrioventricular node blockers for AF are important in reducing morbidity, improving patients' quality of life, and decreasing their risk of tachycardia-induced cardiomyopathy. Guidelines recommend beta-blockers, amiodarone, and nondihydropyridine calcium channel blockers to achieve rate control.[27] In patients without HF, digoxin is not recommended owing to its potential adverse effects. Cardiac glycosides are often used in both AF and HF, despite some studies showing that they increase mortality[38] and the risk of breast cancer.[39,40] Two studies published in 2017 showed that, when used for AF, cardiac glycosides increased patients' risk of breast cancer.[41,42] The Women's Health Initiative, which enrolled 93,676 postmenopausal women from 1994 to 1998 and followed them for 15 years, found that patients with AF had a 5.7% incidence of invasive breast cancer. There was a 19% excess risk of invasive breast cancer with cardiac glycoside use. Independent of AF and other confounders, cardiac glycoside use was strongly associated with incident invasive breast cancer (hazard ratio, 1.68; 95% CI, 1.33–2.12).[41] A meta-analysis of 29 studies published between 1976 and 2016 showed a 33% increase in breast cancer with the use of cardiac glycosides.[42]

Randomized controlled trials assessing the use of catheter ablation for rate control in AF and HF found that it improved patients' quality of life, left ventricular ejection fraction, and functional capacity compared with medical therapy. Although these trials included predominantly male patients, catheter ablation for rate control in AF and HF may be a good alternative treatment in patients intolerant of medications.[43]

Rhythm Control Medications

The recent American College of Cardiology/American Heart Association Task Force on Practice Guidelines and guidelines from the Heart Rhythm Society recommend antiarrhythmic therapy for possible pharmacologic cardioversion.[27] Studies have reported an increase in torsades de pointes, especially when using medications that prolong corrected QT intervals in women compared with men with antiarrhythmic drugs.[35,44] The presence of HF is another risk factor for increased proarrhythmia.

In a 2-year analysis from the AF registry, the use of antiarrhythmic drug therapy was similar in men (28.6%) and women (28.9%).[45] However, women were less likely to undergo electrical cardioversion (26.7% vs 32.4%) and they were less likely to be referred for AF ablation (4.9% vs 5.9%). In contrast, women were more likely to undergo atrioventricular node ablation for rate control of AF (2.9% vs 1.7%). Women were less likely to receive beta-blocker therapy and were more likely to be on digoxin (24.6% vs 22.6%). The Euro Observational Research Programme on Atrial Fibrillation registry reported similar gender differences in treatment patterns.[46] Women with symptomatic AF were more likely to receive rate control therapy alone (33.1%) in comparison with men (26.0%). Women were also less likely to receive electrical cardioversion (18.9% vs 25.5%). Although beta-blocker therapy was similar in men and women (72.5% and 70.0%), women were more likely to be prescribed digoxin (25.0% vs 19.8%).

Rhythm Control via Catheter Ablation of Atrial Fibrillation in Patients with Heart Failure

Guidelines recommend that patients with symptomatic AF uncontrolled by antiarrhythmic drugs or those who cannot tolerate pharmacotherapy should undergo catheter ablation.[27] Although the rates of AF ablation are increasing, women are less likely to undergo catheter ablation than men. Women are also older at the time of AF ablation and are referred for the procedure later compared with men.[47,48]

Some studies have shown that women who undergo AF ablation have a higher procedural complication rate than men.[49] Possible anatomic differences may underlie some sex differences in these outcomes. Studies have suggested that women have a smaller heart size and this factor could influence the outcomes of ablation, which involves catheter manipulation in the heart chambers.[50] The higher procedural complication rate in females may also be due to a greater duration of AF, greater prevalence of nonparoxysmal forms of AF, and higher bleeding complication rates in women compared with men.[51]

Small studies have shown that catheter ablation to restore sinus rhythm in patients with AF and HF leads to an improvement in functional capacity, but no long-term follow-up has been done to show mortality benefit.[52,53] This finding was addressed recently in the Catheter Ablation for Atrial Fibrillation with Heart Failure (CASTLE-AF) study. Patients with AF and HFrEF were randomized to medical therapy or catheter ablation. After a median follow-up of 37.8 months, compared with medical therapy, catheter ablation led to a significantly lower rate of a composite endpoint comprising death from any cause or hospitalization for worsening HF.[54] Unfortunately, trial participants were predominantly male (84%); thus, benefits for women may differ. A longer term (5 years) randomized controlled study to determine mortality benefit from catheter ablation in AF and HF patients is awaiting results.[55]

A recently published study evaluated the impact of female sex on clinical outcomes in the FIRE AND ICE (radiofrequency vs cryoballoon-based therapy) trial of catheter ablation for AF. Female sex was associated with an almost 40% increase in the risk of atrial arrhythmia recurrence and cardiovascular rehospitalization after catheter ablation for AF, suggesting the probable need for a higher level of monitoring for women to decrease the risk of arrhythmia recurrence.[56]

RISK OF COGNITIVE DECLINE WITH ATRIAL FIBRILLATION AND HEART FAILURE

Improved cardiovascular outcomes have led to a growing elderly population. This aging population, coupled with an increase in the incidence of AF and HF, will likely increase patients presenting to their physicians with symptoms of cognitive decline and dementia.[57,58] AF has been consistently shown not only to increase the risk of dementia and cognitive decline, but also to increase the risk of progression to dementia in persons with mild cognitive impairment.[59,60] Biological and physiologic mechanisms that explain this observed association include impaired atrial contraction, reduced cardiac output, low cerebral blood flow, "silent" or "mini" strokes, and increased expression of key molecules implicated in the pathogenesis of Alzheimer's disease.[61,62] Sex differences in cognitive functioning have recently been reported in the Framingham Heart Study, with men who had AF at baseline showing poorer performance in tests of abstract reasoning and executive function compared with women.[63] Epidemiologic studies have reported direct associations between worsening HF and cognitive decline.[60,64–66] Severe atherosclerosis, AF, and HF are all risk factors for dementia.[67]

Relatively little to no literature exists regarding sex differences in cognitive function and decline

Table 3
Factors contributing to poorer outcomes in women with AF and HF compared with men

1. Increased risk of stroke	• Higher use of warfarin • Less likely to receive oral anticoagulants • Less use of aspirin with anticoagulation
2. Higher incidence of HFpEF	• Higher risk of stroke with HFpEF compared with HFrEF
3. Higher use of digoxin	• Increased mortality in some studies • Increased risk of breast cancer
4. Higher risk of procedural complications	• Women are older at the time of AF ablation • Referred for the procedure late after presentation • Greater prevalence of nonparoxysmal forms of AF • Higher bleeding complication rates
5. Lack of data	• Underrepresented in clinical trials
6. Lower socioeconomic status	• Cost of medications and medical care
7. Older age	• More comorbidities

Abbreviations: AF, atrial fibrillation; HF, heart failure; HFpEF, heart failure with preserved ejection fraction; HFrEF, heart failure with reduced ejection fraction.

in persons with HF. A review of the literature[57] noted a dearth of primary data on the association of cognitive impairment and HF, and the studies conducted varied in methodology, making a cross-comparison of potential sex differences in overall cognitive functioning and dementia risk difficult. Because HF is an increasingly important and frequent complication of heart disease, it is imperative that standardized cognitive assessment tools be used in clinical and research studies to assess cognitive functioning in the aging cardiac population.

SUMMARY

Women with both AF and HF are at high risk for stroke, mortality, and other adverse outcomes. Their quality of life may also be negatively impacted. **Table 3** summarizes factors that may contribute to the poorer outcomes seen in women compared with men. Women who present with HF often have HFpEF, but there are no evidence-based therapies for this finding that have been shown to decrease mortality. Women with AF and HFpEF have a higher risk of stroke compared with women with AF and HFrEF. Women have been treated less aggressively with rhythm control and ablation, which may contribute to the higher symptom burden seen in women with concomitant AF and HF compared with men. Digoxin is more often used in women than in men and its use has been associated with an increased risk of breast cancer and in some studies, increased mortality. Compared with warfarin, novel anticoagulants may lead to better stroke outcomes in women, but high costs may prevent their widespread use.

Treatment outcomes of women with AF and HF may improve if an awareness of sex disparities in their treatment increases the use of novel anticoagulants for stroke prevention, decreases the use of digoxin for rate control, and results in more timely and appropriate AF ablation. Risk factor modification may decrease the burden of AF and HF in women and the prevention of both conditions may decrease cognitive impairment in elderly women and men. To determine whether sex differences in therapeutic response exist, it is necessary to ensure adequate representation of women in future randomized trials of interventions for the treatment and prevention of AF, HF, and their associated adverse outcomes.

REFERENCES

1. Braunwald E. Shattuck lecture–cardiovascular medicine at the turn of the millennium: triumphs, concerns, and opportunities. N Engl J Med 1997;337:1360–9.
2. Staerk L, Wang B, Preis SR, et al. Lifetime risk of atrial fibrillation according to optimal, borderline, or elevated levels of risk factors: cohort study based on longitudinal data from the Framingham Heart Study. BMJ 2018;361:k1453.
3. Benjamin EJ, Wolf PA, D'Agostino RB, et al. Impact of atrial fibrillation on the risk of death: the Framingham Heart Study. Circulation 1998;98:946–52.
4. Benjamin EJ, Virani SS, Callaway CW, et al. Heart disease and stroke statistics-2018 update: a report from the American Heart Association. Circulation 2018;137(12):e67–492.
5. Ling LH, Kistler PM, Kalman JM, et al. Comorbidity of atrial fibrillation and heart failure. Nat Rev Cardiol 2016;13:131–47.

6. Kotecha D, Piccini JP. Atrial fibrillation in heart failure: what should we do? Eur Heart J 2015;36: 3250–7.

7. Santhanakrishnan R, Wang N, Larson MG, et al. Atrial fibrillation begets heart failure and vice versa: temporal associations and differences in preserved versus reduced ejection fraction. Circulation 2016; 133:484–92.

8. McManus DD, Hsu G, Sung SH, et al. Atrial fibrillation and outcomes in heart failure with preserved versus reduced left ventricular ejection fraction. J Am Heart Assoc 2013;2:e005694.

9. Wang TJ, Larson MG, Levy D, et al. Temporal relations of atrial fibrillation and congestive heart failure and their joint influence on mortality: the Framingham Heart Study. Circulation 2003;107:2920–5.

10. Khazanie P, Liang L, Qualls LG, et al. Outcomes of Medicare beneficiaries with heart failure and atrial fibrillation. JACC Heart Fail 2014;2:41–8.

11. Emdin CA, Wong CX, Hsiao AJ, et al. Atrial fibrillation as risk factor for cardiovascular disease and death in women compared with men: systematic review and meta-analysis of cohort studies. BMJ 2016; 532:h7013.

12. Chatterjee NA, Chae CU, Kim E, et al. Modifiable risk factors for incident heart failure in atrial fibrillation. JACC Heart Fail 2017;5:552–60.

13. Dryer K, Gajjar M, Narang N, et al. Coronary microvascular dysfunction in patients with heart failure with preserved ejection fraction. Am J Physiol Heart Circ Physiol 2018;314(5):H1033–42.

14. Ebert SN, Liu XK, Woosley RL. Female gender as a risk factor for drug-induced cardiac arrhythmias: evaluation of clinical and experimental evidence. J Womens Health 1998;7:547–57.

15. Rankin SH. Differences in recovery from cardiac surgery: a profile of male and female patients. Heart Lung 1990;19:481–5.

16. Kurt M, Wang J, Torre-Amione G, et al. Left atrial function in diastolic heart failure. Circ Cardiovasc Imaging 2009;2:10–5.

17. Sanders P, Morton JB, Davidson NC, et al. Electrical remodeling of the atria in congestive heart failure: electrophysiological and electroanatomic mapping in humans. Circulation 2003;108:1461–8.

18. Kitzman DW, Little WC, Brubaker PH, et al. Pathophysiological characterization of isolated diastolic heart failure in comparison to systolic heart failure. JAMA 2002;288:2144–50.

19. Pandey A, Omar W, Ayers C, et al. Sex and race differences in lifetime risk of heart failure with preserved ejection fraction and heart failure with reduced ejection fraction. Circulation 2018;137(17): 1814–23.

20. Ho JE, Lyass A, Lee DS, et al. Predictors of new-onset heart failure: differences in preserved versus reduced ejection fraction. Circ Heart Fail 2013;6: 279–86.

21. Regitz-Zagrosek V, Brokat S, Tschope C. Role of gender in heart failure with normal left ventricular ejection fraction. Prog Cardiovasc Dis 2007;49: 241–51.

22. Kitzman DW, Gardin JM, Gottdiener JS, et al, Cardiovascular Health Study Research Group. Importance of heart failure with preserved systolic function in patients > or = 65 years of age. CHS Research Group. Cardiovascular Health Study. Am J Cardiol 2001;87:413–9.

23. Hogg K, Swedberg K, McMurray J. Heart failure with preserved left ventricular systolic function; epidemiology, clinical characteristics, and prognosis. J Am Coll Cardiol 2004;43:317–27.

24. Kotecha D, Lam CS, Van Veldhuisen DJ, et al. Heart failure with preserved ejection fraction and atrial fibrillation: vicious twins. J Am Coll Cardiol 2016; 68:2217–28.

25. Benjamin EJ, Levy D, Vaziri SM, et al. Independent risk factors for atrial fibrillation in a population-based cohort. The Framingham Heart Study. JAMA 1994;271:840–4.

26. Gage BF, Waterman AD, Shannon W, et al. Validation of clinical classification schemes for predicting stroke: results from the National Registry of Atrial Fibrillation. JAMA 2001;285:2864–70.

27. January CT, Wann LS, Alpert JS, et al, American College of Cardiology/American Heart Association Task Force on Practice Guidelines. 2014 AHA/ACC/HRS guideline for the management of patients with atrial fibrillation: a report of the American College of Cardiology/American Heart Association Task Force on Practice Guidelines and the Heart Rhythm Society. J Am Coll Cardiol 2014;64:e1–76.

28. O'Neal WT, Sandesara P, Hammadah M, et al. Gender differences in the risk of adverse outcomes in patients with atrial fibrillation and heart failure with preserved ejection fraction. Am J Cardiol 2017;119: 1785–90.

29. Sullivan RM, Zhang J, Zamba G, et al. Relation of gender-specific risk of ischemic stroke in patients with atrial fibrillation to differences in warfarin anticoagulation control (from AFFIRM). Am J Cardiol 2012; 110:1799–802.

30. Pancholy SB, Sharma PS, Pancholy DS, et al. Meta-analysis of gender differences in residual stroke risk and major bleeding in patients with nonvalvular atrial fibrillation treated with oral anticoagulants. Am J Cardiol 2014;113:485–90.

31. Thompson LE, Maddox TM, Lei L, et al. Sex differences in the use of oral anticoagulants for atrial fibrillation: a report from the National Cardiovascular Data Registry (NCDR(R)) PINNACLE registry. J Am Heart Assoc 2017;6 [pii:e005801].

32. Reddy VY, Doshi SK, Kar S, et al. 5-year outcomes after left atrial appendage closure: from the PREVAIL and PROTECT AF trials. J Am Coll Cardiol 2017;70:2964–75.

33. Hagens VE, Van Veldhuisen DJ, Kamp O, et al. Effect of rate and rhythm control on left ventricular function and cardiac dimensions in patients with persistent atrial fibrillation: results from the RAte Control versus Electrical Cardioversion for Persistent Atrial Fibrillation (RACE) study. Heart Rhythm 2005; 2:19–24.

34. Wyse DG, Waldo AL, DiMarco JP, et al. A comparison of rate control and rhythm control in patients with atrial fibrillation. N Engl J Med 2002;347:1825–33.

35. Rienstra M, Van Veldhuisen DJ, Hagens VE, et al. Gender-related differences in rhythm control treatment in persistent atrial fibrillation: data of the Rate Control Versus Electrical Cardioversion (RACE) study. J Am Coll Cardiol 2005;46:1298–306.

36. Roy D, Talajic M, Nattel S, et al. Rhythm control versus rate control for atrial fibrillation and heart failure. N Engl J Med 2008;358:2667–77.

37. Gillis AM. Atrial fibrillation and ventricular arrhythmias: sex differences in electrophysiology, epidemiology, clinical presentation, and clinical outcomes. Circulation 2017;135:593–608.

38. Pastori D, Farcomeni A, Bucci T, et al. Digoxin treatment is associated with increased total and cardiovascular mortality in anticoagulated patients with atrial fibrillation. Int J Cardiol 2015;180:1–5.

39. Ahern TP, Lash TL, Sorensen HT, et al. Digoxin treatment is associated with an increased incidence of breast cancer: a population-based case-control study. Breast Cancer Res 2008;10:R102.

40. Ahern TP, Tamimi RM, Rosner BA, et al. Digoxin use and risk of invasive breast cancer: evidence from the Nurses' Health Study and meta-analysis. Breast Cancer Res Treat 2014;144:427–35.

41. Wassertheil-Smoller S, McGinn AP, Martin L, et al. The associations of atrial fibrillation with the risks of incident invasive breast and colorectal cancer. Am J Epidemiol 2017;185:372–84.

42. Osman MH, Farrag E, Selim M, et al. Cardiac glycosides use and the risk and mortality of cancer; systematic review and meta-analysis of observational studies. PLoS One 2017;12:e0178611.

43. Zhu M, Zhou X, Cai H, et al. Catheter ablation versus medical rate control for persistent atrial fibrillation in patients with heart failure: a PRISMA-compliant systematic review and meta-analysis of randomized controlled trials. Medicine (Baltimore) 2016;95: e4377.

44. Makkar RR, Fromm BS, Steinman RT, et al. Female gender as a risk factor for torsades de pointes associated with cardiovascular drugs. JAMA 1993;270: 2590–7.

45. Piccini JP, Simon DN, Steinberg BA, et al, Outcomes Registry for Better Informed Treatment of Atrial Fibrillation Investigators and Patients. Differences in clinical and functional outcomes of atrial fibrillation in women and men: two-year results from the ORBIT-AF registry. JAMA Cardiol 2016;1:282–91.

46. Lip GY, Laroche C, Boriani G, et al. Sex-related differences in presentation, treatment, and outcome of patients with atrial fibrillation in Europe: a report from the Euro Observational Research Programme Pilot survey on Atrial Fibrillation. Europace 2015; 17:24–31.

47. Patel N, Deshmukh A, Thakkar B, et al. Gender, race, and health insurance status in patients undergoing catheter ablation for atrial fibrillation. Am J Cardiol 2016;117:1117–26.

48. Sultan A, Luker J, Andresen D, et al. Predictors of atrial fibrillation recurrence after catheter ablation: data from the German ablation registry. Sci Rep 2017;7:16678.

49. Ko D, Rahman F, Martins MA, et al. Atrial fibrillation in women: treatment. Nat Rev Cardiol 2017;14:113–24.

50. Hoyt H, Nazarian S, Alhumaid F, et al. Demographic profile of patients undergoing catheter ablation of atrial fibrillation. J Cardiovasc Electrophysiol 2011; 22:994–8.

51. Patel D, Mohanty P, Di Biase L, et al. Outcomes and complications of catheter ablation for atrial fibrillation in females. Heart Rhythm 2010;7:167–72.

52. Dagres N, Varounis C, Gaspar T, et al. Catheter ablation for atrial fibrillation in patients with left ventricular systolic dysfunction. A systematic review and meta-analysis. J Card Fail 2011;17:964–70.

53. Suman-Horduna I, Roy D, Frasure-Smith N, et al. Quality of life and functional capacity in patients with atrial fibrillation and congestive heart failure. J Am Coll Cardiol 2013;61:455–60.

54. Marrouche NF, Brachmann J, Andresen D, et al. Catheter ablation for atrial fibrillation with heart failure. N Engl J Med 2018;378:417–27.

55. Verma A, Kalman JM, Callans DJ. Treatment of patients with atrial fibrillation and heart failure with reduced ejection fraction. Circulation 2017;135: 1547–63.

56. Kuck KH, Brugada J, Furnkranz A, et al. Impact of female sex on clinical outcomes in the FIRE AND ICE trial of catheter ablation for atrial fibrillation. Circ Arrhythm Electrophysiol 2018;11:e006204.

57. Cannon JA, Moffitt P, Perez-Moreno AC, et al. Cognitive impairment and heart failure: systematic review and meta-analysis. J Card Fail 2017;23:464–75.

58. Aldrugh S, Sardana M, Henninger N, et al. Atrial fibrillation, cognition and dementia: a review. J Cardiovasc Electrophysiol 2017;28:958–65.

59. Forti P, Maioli F, Pisacane N, et al. Atrial fibrillation and risk of dementia in non-demented elderly

subjects with and without mild cognitive impairment. Neurol Res 2006;28:625–9.

60. Di Carlo A, Baldereschi M, Amaducci L, et al. Cognitive impairment without dementia in older people: prevalence, vascular risk factors, impact on disability. The Italian Longitudinal Study on Aging. J Am Geriatr Soc 2000;48:775–82.

61. Kalaria RN. The role of cerebral ischemia in Alzheimer's disease. Neurobiol Aging 2000;21:321–30.

62. Putzke JD, Williams MA, Rayburn BK, et al. The relationship between cardiac function and neuropsychological status among heart transplant candidates. J Card Fail 1998;4:295–303.

63. Nishtala A, Piers RJ, Himali JJ, et al. Atrial fibrillation and cognitive decline in the Framingham Heart Study. Heart Rhythm 2018;15:166–72.

64. Zuccala G, Pedone C, Cesari M, et al. The effects of cognitive impairment on mortality among hospitalized patients with heart failure. Am J Med 2003; 115:97–103.

65. Loncar G, Bozic B, Lepic T, et al. Relationship of reduced cerebral blood flow and heart failure severity in elderly males. Aging Male 2011;14: 59–65.

66. Qiu C, Winblad B, Marengoni A, et al. Heart failure and risk of dementia and Alzheimer disease: a population-based cohort study. Arch Intern Med 2006;166:1003–8.

67. Stefanidis KB, Askew CD, Greaves K, et al. The effect of non-stroke cardiovascular disease states on risk for cognitive decline and dementia: a systematic and meta-analytic review. Neuropsychol Rev 2018; 28(1):1–15.

68. He J, Ogden LG, Bazzano LA, et al. Risk factors for congestive heart failure in US men and women: NHANES I epidemiologic follow-up study. Arch Intern Med 2001;161:996–1002.

69. Magnussen C, Niiranen TJ, Ojeda FM, et al. Sex differences and similarities in atrial fibrillation epidemiology, risk factors, and mortality in community cohorts: results from the BiomarCaRE Consortium (Biomarker for Cardiovascular Risk Assessment in Europe). Circulation 2017;136:1588–97.

Breast Cancer and Heart Failure

Zakaria Almuwaqqat, MD, MPH[a,b,]*, Jane L. Meisel, MD[c,d], Ana Barac, MD, PhD[e,f], Susmita Parashar, MD, MPH, MS[a,d]

KEYWORDS

- Cardiotoxicity • Anthracyclines • Trastuzumab

KEY POINTS

- Heart failure prevention in breast cancer patients starts with optimal management of preexisting cardiovascular risk factors and cardiac surveillance.
- The risk of cardiotoxicity among patients receiving systemic breast cancer therapy varies by age, cardiovascular risk factors, dose and type of chemotherapy, concomitant and sequential use of cardiotoxic agents, exposure to radiotherapy, and history of structural heart disease.
- Multidisciplinary management breast cancer and heart failure management is of utmost importance to ensure best outcomes.

CLINICAL CASE

A 68-year-old woman with stage T4bN1M0, IIIB, breast cancer that was positive for estrogen receptor/progesterone, HER2 negative presented with dyspnea. Her baseline echocardiogram revealed a normal ejection fraction of 60%. She has had neoadjuvant chemotherapy of 4 cycles of dose-dense anthracycline and 3 cycles of dose-dense paclitaxel. One year after treatment, she presented with fatigue, generalized edema, and dyspnea on exertion. Echocardiogram was consistent with diffuse left ventricular (LV) dilatation and reduced ejection fraction 15% to 20%. She was started on heart failure (HF) therapy.

INTRODUCTION

Cancer and cardiovascular disease (CVD) are leading causes of morbidity and mortality in the United States and their co-occurrence is increasingly prevalent.[1] Breast cancer is increasingly a major focus of this association due to high prevalence of the disease and major improvement in survival with modern cancer therapies.[2] Currently there are 3.5 million breast cancer survivors in the United States, with average life expectancy of 90% at 5 years.[3]

CVD competes with breast cancer as the leading cause of death for older women diagnosed with breast cancer.[2] Older women diagnosed with hormone-positive breast cancer are more likely to die from diseases other than cancer, with CVD the most frequent cause.[4,5] Compared with women without a history of breast cancer, older postmenopausal women breast cancer survivors have a higher risk of mortality attributable to CVD, with the risk manifesting itself greater than 7 years after the breast cancer diagnosis. Additionally, patients experience significantly

Disclosure: The authors have nothing to disclose.
[a] Department of Cardiology, Emory University School of Medicine, 1364 Clifton Road, Atlanta, GA 30322, USA; [b] Rollins School of Public Health, Emory University, Atlanta, GA, USA; [c] Department of Hematology and Medical Oncology, Emory University School of Medicine, 1364 Clifton Road, Atlanta, GA 30322, USA; [d] Winship Cancer Institute, Emory University School of Medicine, 1365 Clifton Road Atlanta, GA 30322, USA; [e] MedStar Heart and Vascular Institute, MedStar Washington Hospital Center, 3800 Reservoir Road NW, Washington, DC 20007, USA; [f] Department of Oncology, Georgetown University, 3800 Reservoir Road NW, Washington, DC 20007, USA
* Corresponding author. Department of Medicine, Emory University School of Medicine, 1364 Clifton Road, Atlanta, GA 30328.
E-mail address: zalmuwa@emory.edu

Heart Failure Clin 15 (2019) 65–75
https://doi.org/10.1016/j.hfc.2018.08.007
1551-7136/19/© 2018 Elsevier Inc. All rights reserved.

higher rates of congestive HF (CHF) that persist for 10 years after treatment compared with their age-matched populations.[6]

Breast cancer and CVD share some common risk factors, such as obesity, smoking, excessive alcohol use, unhealthy diet, and physical inactivity,[2] thus opening the door for intervention opportunities to improve outcomes of both illnesses. The Cardiovascular Lifetime Risk Pooling Project demonstrated that individuals with optimal risk factor profiles at age 45 years have a significantly lower lifetime risk of CVD events compared with those with 1 major risk factor (4.1% vs 20.2% among women).[7] Adherence to ideal cardiovascular behavior based on the American Heart Association (AHA) Life's Simple 7 is associated with a trend toward a lower incidence of breast cancer (P for trend = 0.11).[8] Similarly, exercise is also shown to improve vascular endothelial function and exercise capacity in breast cancer and prostate cancer survivors.[9]

Multidisciplinary care that has transformed the prognosis of patients with breast cancer is in increasing need of cardiovascular care providers, to identify and treat preexisting cardiovascular conditions and allow optimal cancer treatment, reduce short-term and long-term risk of HF, and minimize, diagnose, and manage cardiovascular toxicities during and after completion of cancer treatments.[2,10]

This review article summarizes current clinical evidence for cardiovascular and HF risk in patients with breast cancer and evolving primary and secondary prevention strategies during treatment and in survivorship.

CLINICAL CONSIDERATIONS PRIOR TO RECEIPT OF BREAST CANCER TREATMENT
Shared Cardiovascular and Breast Cancer Risk Factors and Common Pathophysiologic Pathways

HF and breast cancer may have a common biological background with overlap in risk factors (**Fig. 1**). Multiple epidemiologic studies have demonstrated that multiple CVD risk factors leading to stage A HF have been associated with the risk of postmenopausal breast cancer. Hypertension has been linked to the increasing incidence of cancer and cancer-related mortality.[11] Similarly, it is well established that obesity is associated with breast cancer risk, in particular the hormone-sensitive tumors.[12,13] Elevated circulating estrogen levels and hormonal production have been implicated as a primary factor in this relationship.[14] Patients with diabetes, obesity, and metabolic syndrome can

have elevated levels of carcinogenic hormonal mediators, which has been linked to the increasing risk of breast cancer, for example, insulinlike growth factor 1 and estrogen.[14] Moreover, adipokines synthesized in adipose tissue may influence breast tumorigenesis by having an impact on both circulating and locally produced levels of these proteins.[15]

Additionally, patients with metabolic syndrome may have a higher inflammatory burden, which may increase the risk of breast cancer.[16] Thus, it is plausible that hypertension, diabetes, obesity, and metabolic syndrome could lead to adverse cardiac and vascular events while simultaneously increasing the risk of carcinogenesis. It is prudent that patients with CVD risk factors undergo an enhanced cardiac surveillance and prevention program. This was supported by recent evidence that adoption of CVD prevention health behaviors is associated with lower cancer incidence and aggressive CVD risk prevention is associated with a reduction in the lifetime risk of cancer.[8,17]

Breast Cancer Systemic Therapies as Risk Factors for Cardiac Dysfunction

Anthracyclines and trastuzumab are the most commonly used cardiotoxic breast cancer therapy. Anthracyclines are the most well-known cardiotoxic chemotherapy used in humans and for decades have been an integral component of systemic breast cancer treatment. Anthracyclines are potent inhibitors of topoisomerase and thus DNA function, leading to dose-related cardiotoxicity. Cardiotoxicity may range from asymptomatic LV systolic dysfunction to clinical and overt HF, which is the most common reason for limiting doxorubicin or epirubicin and/or using nonanthracycline regimens.[18–20] Recent studies have reported that overall anthracycline use in breast cancer treatment has significantly declined over time, although it remains the treatment of choice for select subtypes, such as triple-negative breast cancer.[21] Contemporary anthracycline-containing regimens for early (nonmetastatic) breast cancer typically include a cumulative dose of 240 mg/m^2 of doxorubicin (or similar 600 mg/m^2 of epirubicin), which is considered low based on the early studies that first established linear relationship of cardiac dysfunction with doxorubicin doses above 300 mg/m^2.[22,23]

Multiple studies suggest that anthracycline-based adjuvant chemotherapy carries a substantial long-term risk of HF lasting for years, especially for women older than 65 years of age.[24] Although adjuvant trials typically report only symptomatic

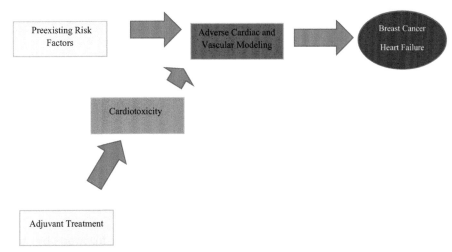

Fig. 1. Factors implicated in the generation of breast cancer and HF.

cardiac events, recent prospective studies report frequent subclinical LV dysfunction in approximately 10% to 50% of patients receiving anthracycline-based therapy.[25] The long-term consequences of subclinical LV dysfunction are not known, although this could leave patients more susceptible to further adverse cardiac remodeling, leading to clinical HF. Biological mechanisms underlying chemotherapy-associated cardiac dysfunction remain to be fully understood. Generation of reactive oxygen species (ROS) was believed to play a central role but recent studies have reported that ROS scavengers failed to prevent cardiac toxicity[26] caused by doxorubicin. Additionally, cardiomyocyte-specific deletion of Top2b (encoding topoisomerase-IIβ) protects cardiomyocytes from doxorubicin-induced DNA double-strand breaks and may be responsible for defective mitochondrial biogenesis.[27] Earlier exposure to anthracyclines may promote adverse cardiac modeling in the absence of drug as evidenced by mitochondrial DNA alterations, superoxide, and respiratory chain dysfunction accumulation in the absence of the anthracyclines.[28]

Trastuzumab is a human epidermal growth factor receptor 2 (HER2) antagonist that blocks the overexpressed signaling pathway in HER2-positive breast cancers that constitute approximately 20% of all breast cancer cases. Trastuzumab has dramatically improved outcomes in patients with HER2-positive metastatic breast cancer; based on the evidence that the addition of trastuzumab to doxorubicin-containing chemotherapy was shown to markedly improved overall survival.[29] Approximately one-third (27%) of patients receiving trastuzumab and doxorubicin developed cardiomyopathy and HF.[30] This has led to major safety improvement measures,

including separate administration of anthracyclines and trastuzumab and close LV ejection fraction (LVEF) surveillance with recommended treatment cessation or hold if significant (>10%) LVEF decline is identified. There are some discrepancies, however, in recommendations across guidelines, reflecting continuous evolution of the cardiovascular safety monitoring of trastuzumab.[30]

Pertuzumab is a monoclonal antibody used in combination with trastuzumab and docetaxel for the treatment of metastatic HER2-positive breast cancer; it also is used in the same combination as a neoadjuvant in early HER2-positive breast cancer. Studies regarding potential cardiac effects of dual HER-2 blockade with trastuzumab and pertuzumab are conflicting.[31,32]

Breast Cancer Treatment Selection for Patients with and Without Left Ventricular Dysfunction

Before initiation of therapy, a thorough patient history and physical examination should be taken that include determination of baseline cardiovascular risk.[33] Selection of breast cancer treatment is based on a complex model, including patient factors (age, comorbidities, functional status, and patient preference) and tumor factors (lymph node involvement, histologic grade, genomic tests when available, and HER2 status and hormone receptor status). Often, clinical profile and preexisting risk factors dictate certain aspects of treatment (**Fig. 2**).

Depending on the severity of LV dysfunction and/or presence of clinical HF (stages C and D), patients undergoing adjuvant or neoadjuvant chemotherapy may not receive anthracycline-based regimens in situations where this otherwise

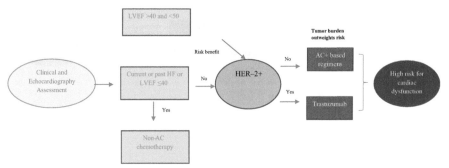

Fig. 2. Treatment selection for patients with breast cancer in patients receiving systemic therapy. AC, anthracycline agents.

is indicated. For anthracycline-based regimens, patients with stage C or stage B HF with LV dysfunction and reduced ejection fraction to 40% or less are usually prohibited from anthracycline-based regimens. Those with LVEF 40% to 50% can be considered for anthracycline regimens based on tumor burden and if the benefits outweigh risks of cardiac dysfunction. Although angiotensin-converting enzyme inhibitor (ACEI)/angiotensin receptor blocker (ARB) and β-blockade initiation among these patients is a common clinical practice, there is no evidence to support the protective effects of ACEIs/ARBs and β-blockade initiation in those patients.

Table 1 displays potential myocardial dysfunction risks of breast cancer systemic therapy. Although anthracycline is usually used on day 1 of 21 for 4 to 6 cycles, trustuzumab and pertuzumab are usually used for longer period of 52 weeks, at least for early breast cancer therapy, and more for metastatic breast cancer. Optimal preventive management of cardiotoxicity requires a multidisciplinary approach with close collaboration between the treating oncologist, internist, and cardiologist; primary prevention starts with the proper selection of breast cancer systemic treatment. According to the American Society of Clinical oncology clinical practice guideline,[33] patients who receive any of the following are considered high-risk of cardiotoxicity:

- High-dose anthracycline (eg, doxorubicin <250 mg/m^2, epirubicin <600 mg/m^2)
- High-dose radiotherapy (<30 Gy), where the heart is in the treatment field.
- Lower-dose anthracycline (eg, doxorubicin ≥250 mg/m^2, epirubicin ≥600 mg/m^2) in combination with lower- dose radiotherapy (≥30 Gy), where the heart is in the treatment field.
- Treatment with lower-dose anthracycline (eg, doxorubicin ≥250 mg/m^2, epirubicin ≥600 mg/m^2) followed by trastuzumab (sequential therapy)
- Treatment with lower-dose anthracycline (eg, doxorubicin <250 mg/m^2, epirubicin <600 mg/m^2) followed by trastuzumab
- Treatment with lower-dose anthracycline (eg, doxorubicin <250 mg/m^2, epirubicin <600 mg/m^2) or trastuzumab alone and presence of any of the following risk factors:
  ○ Multiple cardiovascular risk factors (at least 2 risk factors), including smoking, hypertension, diabetes, dyslipidemia, and obesity
  ○ Older age (at least 60 years) at cancer treatment
  ○ Compromised cardiac function (for example, borderline LVEF [50% to 55%], history of myocardial infarction, or moderate valvular heart disease) at any time before or during treatment.

It is also important to acknowledge that patients with breast cancer and preexisting cardiovascular risk factors are at higher risk for LV dysfunction, as demonstrated by multiple studies showing that hypertension, smoking history, and diabetes are independent predictors of cardiac toxicity in patients who were exposed to trastuzumab and/or anthracycline use.[34,35] Thus, appropriate management for these risk factors should take into account the risk of LV dysfunction to chemotherapy, which may necessitate the maximization of cardiac protection among this group of patients.

Primary Prevention Studies and Management of Preexisting Cardiovascular Disease Risk

Primary prevention strategies for HF in patients receiving systemic breast cancer treatment starts with risk stratification and potential treatment in high-risk patients. **Table 2** summarizes the most recent studies evaluating cardioprotective therapies in reducing the incidence of cardiac toxicity.

Table 1
Potential myocardial dysfunction risks of systemic breast cancer systemic therapy

Systemic Therapy	Duration and Frequency	Common Cardiomyopathy Risks	Comments
Anthracyclines	• Day 1 of 21 per cycle for 4–6 cycles	• Range from LV dysfunction to clinical HF	• Overt HF • Pericarditis/ myocarditis • Cardiomyopathy— cumulative toxicity and dose-related toxicity
Taxanes	• Early breast cancer: every 3 wk for 4 cycles • Metastatic breast cancer: every 3 wk until disease progression or unacceptable toxicity	• Cardiac toxicity is uncommon.	• HF • Myocardial ischemia
HER-2–directed therapies			
Trastuzumab	• Early breast cancer: every 3 wk for 52 wk • Metastatic breast cancer: weekly until disease progression or unacceptable toxicity	• Reversible LV dysfunction	• HF is more common in sequential therapy with anthracycline. • Usually administered in combination with pertuzumab.
Pertuzumab	• Early breast cancer: every 3 wk for 52 wk • Metastatic breast cancer: every 3 wk until disease progression or unacceptable toxicity	• Reversible LV dysfunction	• HF is more common in sequential therapy with anthracycline. • Usually administered in combination with trastuzumab
ER + directed therapies			
Tamoxifen	• Daily for 5–10 y • With or without aromatase inhibitors	• Venous thrombosis	
Aromatase inhibitors	• Daily for 5–10 y	• Uncommon	• Increased risk for cardiovascular adverse events—debatable
Radiotherapy			
Whole-breast radiation therapy	• 40–42.5 Gy for 3–5 wk vs 45–50 Gy for 4.5–5 wk	• Cardiac toxicity risk usually after 10 y of exposure • Radiotherapy safety is unknown when combined with cardiotoxic agents	• HF • Sudden cardiac death • Diffuse intimal hyperplasia of coronary arteries/left main stenosis • Pericardial constriction and thickening of the pericardium and pericardial effusion • Valvular heart disease

There is evidence that ACEIs and ARBs can protect against anthracycline-related cardiac dysfunction in high-risk patients defined by an increased troponin I value.[36] Similarly, treatment with candesartan provided protection against early decline in global LV function in patients treated for early breast cancer with adjuvant anthracycline-containing regimens (with or without trastuzumab and radiation).[37] Certain β-adrenergic receptors blocking agents have also been

Table 2
Clinical trials evaluating potential cardioprotective strategies for breast cancer patients receiving cardiotoxic therapies

Study	Population	Treatment Aims	Primary Endpoint	Outcome	Follow-up Period	Notes
Seicean et al,[42] 2012	201 (breast cancer received anthracycline-based regime ns)	Uninterrupted statin vs propensity scores matched controls	New-onset HF requiring hospitalization	Incident HF and cancer-related mortality were significantly lower in the statin group	2.6 y ± SD 1.7	First study to show a protective effect for statin
Cardinale et al,[36] 2006	473 (breast, lymphoma, and sarcoma) Anthracycline-based regimens	Enalapril vs no treatment	Cardiotoxicity (absolute fall >10% points to below normal limit of 50%)	Cardiotoxicity incidence Control 25/58 (43%) Enalapril 0/56 (0%)	12 mo from randomization	Only high-risk patients with CTnI >70 ng/L after chemotherapy were randomized.
Gulati et al,[37] 2016	130 (breast cancer) Anthracycline-based regimens with or without trustuzumab	Candesartan vs metoprolol vs candesartan + metoprolol	Change in LVEF on completion of adjuvant therapy	Mean LVEF % point reduction (95% CI) Placebo: 2.6 (1.5–3.8) Candesartan: 0.8 (−0.04–1.9) Metoprolol: 1.6 (0.4–2.8)	3–5 mo for patients receiving anthracycline only. 15 mo for 22% of patients receiving additional trastuzumab	PRADA study: cardiac MRI allowed detection of small changes in LVEF
Kaya et al,[40] 2013	45 (breast cancer) Anthracycline-based regimens	Nebivolol vs placebo	Change in LVEF from baseline	LVEF change pre/post placebo: 66.6%/57.5% Nebivolol: 65.6%/63.8%	6 mo from randomization	N-terminal pro-brain natriuretic peptide was increased in the placebo group but unchanged in the nebivolol group.
Kalay et al,[39] 2006	50 (breast, lymphoma, other) Anthracycline-based regimens	Carvedilol vs placebo	Change in LVEF from baseline	LVEF change pre/post placebo: 68.9%/52.3% Carvedilol:70.5%/69.7%	6 mo from randomization	High cumulative anthracycline doses (>700 mg/m² epirubicin)

Study	N	Intervention	Outcome	Results	Timepoint	Comments
Pituskin et al,[38] 2017	33 (breast cancer receiving trustuzumab)	Perindopril vs bisoprolol vs placebo	Change in LV volume and LVEF	No difference in the primary outcome. (LV end-diastolic volume was increased in perindopril patients by 7 ± 14 mL/m², in bisoprolol patients by 8 mL $\pm$ 9 mL/m², and in placebo patients by 4 ± 11 mL/m² ($P = .36$)	52 wk	MANTICORE study: decline in LVEF was attenuated in bisoprolol-treated patients ($-1 \pm 5\%$) relative to the perindopril ($-3 \pm 4\%$) and placebo ($-5 \pm 5\%$) groups ($P = .001$)
Avila et al,[41] 2018	200 HER-2 negative breast cancer and normal LVEF Anthracycline-based regimens	Carvedilol	LVEF reduction	No difference In LVEF reduction incidence or BNP levels	6 mo from randomization	Significant decrease in troponin levels and reduced diastolic dysfunction incidence in carvedilol group

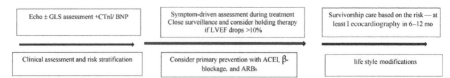

Fig. 3. Cardiac protection during different phases of breast cancer therapies.

shown to have some protective effects from cardiac toxicity. For example, in an analysis of the multidisciplinary approach to novel therapies in cardio-oncology research (MANTICORE) trial that compared perindopril versus bisoprolol versus placebo, trastuzumab-mediated decline in LVEF was attenuated in bisoprolol-treated patients ($-1 \pm 5\%$) relative to the perindopril ($-3 \pm 4\%$) and placebo ($-5 \pm 5\%$) groups ($P = .001$).[38] In the contrary, another study that randomized subjects to placebo versus nebivolol and carvedilol, respectively, found no significant effects on LVEF change pretreatment and post-treatment compared with placebo.[39,40] In a recent analysis of carvedilol compared with placebo among subjects receiving anthracycline therapy,[41] there were no differences noted in changes of LVEF or brain natriuretic peptide (BNP) between groups; however, a significant difference was noticed between groups in troponin levels over time, with lower levels in the carvedilol group ($P = .003$), indicating a possible cardioprotective effect. Additionally, a lower incidence of diastolic dysfunction was noted in the carvedilol group ($P = .039$). These trials were limited, however, by a shorter duration of follow-up and small sample sizes. Statin use among patients with breast cancer receiving anthracycline is associated with significantly reduced incidence of HF compared with their propensity-matched controls.[42]

CLINICAL MANAGEMENT OF HEART FAILURE DURING BREAST CANCER TREATMENT
Defining Cardiac Dysfunction in Breast Cancer Patients Receiving Systemic Therapy

The current definition of cardiac toxicity used by clinicians to make a decision regarding treatment continuation is "a decrease in LVEF greater than 10%, to a value below the lower limit of normal (LVEF <50%)."[43] This definition has evolved over years, however, because a change in LVEF could constitute a late manifestation and potentially irreversible damage. Additionally, although changes in LVEF remain a key parameter in clinical decision making, a review of breast cancer clinical trials showed that a significant variability exists in the definition of cardiac dysfunction used in clinical trials.[44] This has led the current research to focus on

identifying novel echocardiographic markers of cardiac toxicity using speckle-tracking technique to evaluate myocardial strain.[45,46] For example, in breast cancer patients, a decrease in global longitudinal strain (GLS) in a patient receiving doxorubicin and trastuzumab has been shown to predict subsequent LV dysfunction. The American Society of Echocardiography expert consensus document on multimodality imaging of patients undergoing cancer treatment recommends inclusion of GLS and cardiac troponin (CTnI) in risk stratification of patients before and during treatment with anthracyclines or trastuzumab.[45]

More recent trials endpoints provide new data about cardiac serum biomarkers like BNPs and CTnI, LV remodeling, and myocardial strain as potential tools for risk stratification. Studies have shown that CTnI may detect cardiotoxicity at a preclinical phase, long before any reduction in LVEF has occurred, in breast cancer patients receiving chemotherapy.[47,48] Furthermore, the timing of troponin release during and after chemotherapy was found predictive of cardiac events among 703 subjects with breast cancer in the 3 years thereafter.[49]

Strategies of Cardiac Surveillance

At present, baseline assessment of LV function is indicated for all patients starting potentially cardiotoxic therapies, including anthracyclines or HER2 targeted therapies (**Fig. 3**). Recognition of abnormalities in these echocardiographic parameters should prompt initiation of effective cardiac therapies with reassessment of LV function within several weeks. Once a patient has started treatment, cardiovascular testing usually is symptom driven but also depends on the baseline cardiovascular risk profile and the specific cancer treatment regimen. The frequency of LVEF assessment in asymptomatic patients has been debated. For anthracycline-based regimens, imaging is not indicated for patients receiving low-dose doxorubicin regimen (less than 250 mg/m^2) no further routine imaging during treatment is indicated, whereas imaging is recommended for patients receiving a cumulative dose of anthracyclines greater than 250 mg/m^2 prior to each additional dose of 50 mg/m^2.[33] Asymptomatic subjects who are considered at high risk of cardiotoxicity should receive repeat imaging at completion and in 6 months to 12 months afterward.

For HER2-targeted therapy, routine surveillance is usually performed every 3 months during 1 year of treatment in an early breast cancer setting or lifelong in a metastatic setting. At completion of therapy, cardiac surveillance is typically done for only those who had received HER-2 targeted therapy with prior anthracycline exposure.[50]

Patients Developing Cardiac Dysfunction During Treatment

Patients developing HF during systemic treatment should be treated according to guidelines from the American College of Cardiology/AHA.[51] Involvement of a cardio-oncologist is recommended when clinical HF or a decline of LVEF is noted during chemotherapy because careful decision making is required with respect to further exposure to cardiotoxic cancer treatment. Depending on the gain from further cancer therapy, it is sometimes possible to continue treatment with the support of ACEIs and β-blockade. A recent study has found that of 226 patients who developed cardiotoxicity after anthracycline-based chemotherapy and received treatment with ACEIs and β-blocker in combination, 11% had complete recovery of LVEF, 18% had no recovery, and the remainder exhibited partial LVEF recovery to baseline over a period of 5-year echocardiographic follow-up.[36,38]

Safety of HER2 Targeted Therapy in Patients with HER2-Positive Breast Cancer and reduced LV Dysfunction trial (SAFE-HEaRt) will provide needed safety data about initiation and/or continuation of HER2 agents (trastuzumab, pertuzumab, and T-DM1) in patients with mild LV dysfunction.[52]

Breast Cancer Survivorship and Heart Failure Risk Management

The development of novel oncologic therapies that improve cancer-free and overall survival rates but may cause treatment-associated LV dysfunction highlights the need for continual collaboration between oncology and cardiology teams during cancer treatment continuum, including cancer survivorship.[53] Recent data in childhood cancer survivors point to a some degree of synergism between exposure to anthracycline-based chemotherapy and cardiovascular risk factors with regards to HF risk.[54] Developing hearts may be particularly susceptible and remain at increased risk of heart failure decades after therapy, and ongoing research illustrates potential mechanisms that may be applicable in adult population as well.[55]

Prevalence of mild asymptomatic LV dysfunction among breast cancer survivors has not been systematically studied and LVEF assessment after completion of cancer treatment has not been a part of oncology clinical practice. Recent American Society of Clinical Oncology cardiac dysfunction guidelines recommend a single echocardiogram 6 months to 12 months after completion of anthracycline therapy in high-risk asymptomatic patients.[33] Similarly, the National Comprehensive Cancer Network guidelines recommend consideration of an echocardiogram in patients who received low-dose anthracycline and have 2 or more cardiovascular risk factors. Cardiology consensus statements recommend more frequent (at the completion of treatment and 6 months after) or longer follow-up (at 1 years and 5 years), albeit recognizing lack of data regarding frequency and duration of LVEF monitoring in cancer survivors.

Prevention of overt HF in breast cancer survivors remains an important research and clinical collaboration opportunity. Data from cardiovascular cohorts point to increased risk of progression to HF and cardiovascular mortality in individuals with asymptomatic LV dysfunction.[34] Intervention studies focused on cardiovascular, HF, and oncology outcomes are needed to guide clinical practice.

SUMMARY

HF developing during or after breast cancer therapy is a growing heath concern that should be addressed in multidisciplinary settings involving close collaboration between cardiology and oncology to insure the best possible survival and quality of life. Optimal preventive efforts should start with proper risk stratification and careful selection of chemotherapy regimens combined with management of underlying risk factors. The evidence for potential need of using cardiac protection therapy is evolving and so is the definition of cardiac toxicity allowing earlier detection of subtle LV changes and promoting safe and effective use of chemotherapy for subjects with breast cancer while ensuring the best outcomes of their overall health status.

REFERENCES

1. Hung WW, Ross JS, Boockvar KS, et al. Recent trends in chronic disease, impairment and disability among older adults in the United States. BMC Geriatr 2011;11:47.
2. Mehta LS, Watson KE, Barac A, et al, American Heart Association Cardiovascular Disease in Women and

Special Populations Committee of the Council on Clinical Cardiology; Council on Cardiovascular and Stroke Nursing; and Council on Quality of Care and Outcomes Research. Cardiovascular disease and breast cancer: where these entities intersect: a scientific statement from the American Heart Association. Circulation 2018;137:e30–66.

3. Miller KD, Siegel RL, Lin CC, et al. Cancer treatment and survivorship statistics, 2016. CA Cancer J Clin 2016;66:271–89.

4. Patnaik JL, Byers T, DiGuiseppi C, et al. Cardiovascular disease competes with breast cancer as the leading cause of death for older females diagnosed with breast cancer: a retrospective cohort study. Breast Cancer Res 2011;13:R64.

5. Jones LW, Haykowsky MJ, Swartz JJ, et al. Early breast cancer therapy and cardiovascular injury. J Am Coll Cardiol 2007;50:1435–41.

6. Pinder MC, Duan Z, Goodwin JS, et al. Congestive heart failure in older women treated with adjuvant anthracycline chemotherapy for breast cancer. J Clin Oncol 2007;25:3808–15.

7. Berry JD, Dyer A, Cai X, et al. Lifetime risks of cardiovascular disease. N Engl J Med 2012;366: 321–9.

8. Rasmussen-Torvik LJ, Shay CM, Abramson JG, et al. Ideal cardiovascular health is inversely associated with incident cancer: the atherosclerosis risk in communities study. Circulation 2013;127:1270–5.

9. Beaudry RI, Liang Y, Boyton ST, et al. Meta-analysis of exercise training on vascular endothelial function in cancer survivors. Integr Cancer Ther 2018;17(2): 192–9.

10. Barac A, Murtagh G, Carver JR, et al. Cardiovascular health of patients with cancer and cancer survivors: a roadmap to the next level. J Am Coll Cardiol 2015;65:2739–46.

11. Stocks T, Van Hemelrijck M, Manjer J, et al. Blood pressure and risk of cancer incidence and mortality in the metabolic syndrome and cancer project. Hypertension 2012;59:802–10.

12. Cleary MP, Grossmann ME. Minireview: obesity and breast cancer: the estrogen connection. Endocrinology 2009;150:2537–42.

13. Rosato V, Bosetti C, Talamini R, et al. Metabolic syndrome and the risk of breast cancer in postmenopausal women. Ann Oncol 2011;22:2687–92.

14. Lorincz AM, Sukumar S. Molecular links between obesity and breast cancer. Endocr Relat Cancer 2006;13:279–92.

15. Ray A, Nkhata KJ, Cleary MP. Effects of leptin on human breast cancer cell lines in relationship to estrogen receptor and HER2 status. Int J Oncol 2007;30: 1499–509.

16. Yao X, Huang J, Zhong H, et al. Targeting interleukin-6 in inflammatory autoimmune diseases and cancers. Pharmacol Ther 2014;141:125–39.

17. Kushi LH, Doyle C, McCullough M, et al, American Cancer Society 2010 Nutrition and Physical Activity Guidelines Advisory Committee. American Cancer Society Guidelines on nutrition and physical activity for cancer prevention: reducing the risk of cancer with healthy food choices and physical activity. CA Cancer J Clin 2012;62: 30–67.

18. Cardinale D, Colombo A, Lamantia G, et al. Anthracycline-induced cardiomyopathy: clinical relevance and response to pharmacologic therapy. J Am Coll Cardiol 2010;55:213–20.

19. Lotrionte M, Biondi-Zoccai G, Abbate A, et al. Review and meta-analysis of incidence and clinical predictors of anthracycline cardiotoxicity. Am J Cardiol 2013;112:1980–4.

20. Jensen BV. Cardiotoxic consequences of anthracycline-containing therapy in patients with breast cancer. Semin Oncol 2006;33:S15–21.

21. Giordano SH, Lin YL, Kuo YF, et al. Decline in the use of anthracyclines for breast cancer. J Clin Oncol 2012;30:2232–9.

22. Von Hoff DD, Layard MW, Basa P, et al. Risk factors for doxorubicin-induced congestive heart failure. Ann Intern Med 1979;91:710–7.

23. Swain SM, Whaley FS, Ewer MS. Congestive heart failure in patients treated with doxorubicin: a retrospective analysis of three trials. Cancer 2003;97: 2869–79.

24. Doyle JJ, Neugut AI, Jacobson JS, et al. Chemotherapy and cardiotoxicity in older breast cancer patients: a population-based study. J Clin Oncol 2005; 23:8597–605.

25. Perez EA, Suman VJ, Davidson NE, et al. Effect of doxorubicin plus cyclophosphamide on left ventricular ejection fraction in patients with breast cancer in the North Central Cancer Treatment Group N9831 Intergroup Adjuvant Trial. J Clin Oncol 2004;22: 3700–4.

26. Martin E, Thougaard AV, Grauslund M, et al. Evaluation of the topoisomerase II-inactive bisdioxopiperazine ICRF-161 as a protectant against doxorubicin-induced cardiomyopathy. Toxicology 2009;255: 72–9.

27. Zhang S, Liu X, Bawa-Khalfe T, et al. Identification of the molecular basis of doxorubicin-induced cardiotoxicity. Nat Med 2012;18:1639–42.

28. Lebrecht D, Setzer B, Ketelsen UP, et al. Time-dependent and tissue-specific accumulation of mtDNA and respiratory chain defects in chronic doxorubicin cardiomyopathy. Circulation 2003;108: 2423–9.

29. Slamon DJ, Leyland-Jones B, Shak S, et al. Use of chemotherapy plus a monoclonal antibody against HER2 for metastatic breast cancer that overexpresses HER2. N Engl J Med 2001;344: 783–92.

30. Seidman A, Hudis C, Pierri MK, et al. Cardiac dysfunction in the trastuzumab clinical trials experience. J Clin Oncol 2002;20:1215–21.

31. Yu AF, Manrique C, Pun S, et al. Cardiac safety of paclitaxel plus trastuzumab and pertuzumab in patients with HER2-positive metastatic breast cancer. Oncologist 2016;21:418–24.

32. van Ramshorst MS, van Werkhoven E, Honkoop AH, et al, Dutch Breast Cancer Research Group. Toxicity of dual HER2-blockade with pertuzumab added to anthracycline versus non-anthracycline containing chemotherapy as neoadjuvant treatment in HER2-positive breast cancer: the TRAIN-2 study. Breast 2016;29:153–9.

33. Armenian SH, Lacchetti C, Barac A, et al. Prevention and monitoring of cardiac dysfunction in survivors of adult cancers: American Society of Clinical Oncology clinical practice guideline. J Clin Oncol 2017;35:893–911.

34. Wang TJ, Evans JC, Benjamin EJ, et al. Natural history of asymptomatic left ventricular systolic dysfunction in the community. Circulation 2003; 108:977–82.

35. Wadhwa D, Fallah-Rad N, Grenier D, et al. Trastuzumab mediated cardiotoxicity in the setting of adjuvant chemotherapy for breast cancer: a retrospective study. Breast Cancer Res Treat 2009; 117:357–64.

36. Cardinale D, Colombo A, Sandri MT, et al. Prevention of high-dose chemotherapy-induced cardiotoxicity in high-risk patients by angiotensin-converting enzyme inhibition. Circulation 2006;114:2474–81.

37. Gulati G, Heck SL, Ree AH, et al. Prevention of cardiac dysfunction during adjuvant breast cancer therapy (PRADA): a 2 x 2 factorial, randomized, placebo-controlled, double-blind clinical trial of candesartan and metoprolol. Eur Heart J 2016;37: 1671–80.

38. Pituskin E, Mackey JR, Koshman S, et al. Multidisciplinary approach to novel therapies in cardio-oncology research (MANTICORE 101-Breast): a randomized trial for the prevention of trastuzumab-associated cardiotoxicity. J Clin Oncol 2017;35: 870–7.

39. Kalay N, Basar E, Ozdogru I, et al. Protective effects of carvedilol against anthracycline-induced cardiomyopathy. J Am Coll Cardiol 2006;48:2258–62.

40. Kaya MG, Ozkan M, Gunebakmaz O, et al. Protective effects of nebivolol against anthracycline-induced cardiomyopathy: a randomized control study. Int J Cardiol 2013;167:2306–10.

41. Avila MS, Ayub-Ferreira SM, de Barros Wanderley Junior MR, et al. Carvedilol for prevention of chemotherapy related cardiotoxicity: the CECCY trial. J Am Coll Cardiol 2018;71(20):2281–90.

42. Seicean S, Seicean A, Plana JC, et al. Effect of statin therapy on the risk for incident heart failure in patients with breast cancer receiving anthracycline chemotherapy: an observational clinical cohort study. J Am Coll Cardiol 2012;60:2384–90.

43. Groarke JD, Nohria A. Anthracycline cardiotoxicity: a new paradigm for an old classic. Circulation 2015;131:1946–9.

44. Ohad Oren MO. Clinical trials of cardiotoxicity in breast cancer. J Am Coll Cardiol 2017;69.

45. Sawaya H, Sebag IA, Plana JC, et al. Assessment of echocardiography and biomarkers for the extended prediction of cardiotoxicity in patients treated with anthracyclines, taxanes, and trastuzumab. Circ Cardiovasc Imaging 2012;5:596–603.

46. Thavendiranathan P, Poulin F, Lim KD, et al. Use of myocardial strain imaging by echocardiography for the early detection of cardiotoxicity in patients during and after cancer chemotherapy: a systematic review. J Am Coll Cardiol 2014;63:2751–68.

47. Cardinale D, Sandri MT, Martinoni A, et al. Myocardial injury revealed by plasma troponin I in breast cancer treated with high-dose chemotherapy. Ann Oncol 2002;13:710–5.

48. Curigliano G, Cardinale D, Dent S, et al. Cardiotoxicity of anticancer treatments: epidemiology, detection, and management. CA Cancer J Clin 2016;66: 309–25.

49. Cardinale D, Sandri MT, Colombo A, et al. Prognostic value of troponin I in cardiac risk stratification of cancer patients undergoing high-dose chemotherapy. Circulation 2004;109:2749–54.

50. Dang CT, Yu AF, Jones LW, et al. Cardiac surveillance guidelines for trastuzumab-containing therapy in early-stage breast cancer: getting to the heart of the matter. J Clin Oncol 2016;34:1030–3.

51. Yancy CW, Jessup M, Bozkurt B, et al. 2017 ACC/AHA/HFSA focused update of the 2013 ACCF/AHA guideline for the management of heart failure: a report of the American College of Cardiology/American Heart Association Task Force on clinical practice guidelines and the Heart Failure Society of America. Circulation 2017;136:e137–61.

52. Lynce F, Barac A, Tan MT, et al. SAFE-HEaRt: rationale and design of a pilot study investigating cardiac safety of HER2 targeted therapy in patients with HER2-positive breast cancer and reduced left ventricular function. Oncologist 2017;22: 518–25.

53. Parashar S. Building bridges: the emerging field of cardio-oncology. Future Cardiol 2015;11:377–82.

54. Armstrong GT, Oeffinger KC, Chen Y, et al. Modifiable risk factors and major cardiac events among adult survivors of childhood cancer. J Clin Oncol 2013;31:3673–80.

55. Bhatia S, Armenian SH, Armstrong GT, et al. Collaborative research in childhood cancer survivorship: the current landscape. J Clin Oncol 2015;33: 3055–64.

Valvular Heart Disease and Heart Failure in Women

Daniela R. Crousillat, MD[a], Malissa J. Wood, MD[b],*

KEYWORDS

- Women • Valvular heart disease • Heart failure • Aortic stenosis • Mitral regurgitation
- Tricuspid regurgitation

KEY POINTS

- Valvular heart disease (VHD) and heart failure (HF) remain important causes of cardiovascular disease among women in the United States.
- Sex differences exist in the epidemiology, diagnosis, treatment, and outcomes among the most common VHDs including mitral regurgitation, aortic stenosis, and tricuspid regurgitation.
- Severe VHD in pregnancy, specifically left-sided stenotic valvular lesions, is associated with HF and adverse cardiovascular complications.

INTRODUCTION

Heart failure (HF) is more prevalent in women compared with men and remains a leading cause of morbidity and mortality in the United States. Currently, 3 million women live with HF, and the prevalence is projected to continue to increase.[1] Valvular heart disease (VHD) is present among 2.5% of the US population and can be the primary driver of ventricular dysfunction and HF due to detrimental hemodynamic loading, or it can often develop secondary to existing ventricular dysfunction. Mitral regurgitation (MR) and aortic stenosis (AS) are the most common valvular lesions among men and women in the United States.[2] Despite their similar prevalence among both sexes, important sex differences exist in the epidemiology, diagnosis, treatment, and outcomes.

Women with severe MR have unique valvular pathologic condition, present with more advanced disease, and suffer from delayed referral for surgical interventions with less favorable outcomes.[3–5] In addition, because of smaller body surface area (BSA), women are at risk for delayed treatment due to the absence of indexing of echocardiographic parameters currently recommended by societal guidelines for referral to surgical intervention.[6] Women with degenerative AS have unique valvular pathophysiology requiring gender-specific considerations for the accurate diagnosis of severe AS, including the recognition of paradoxic low-flow, low-gradient (LF-LG) AS, a more prevalent but higher-risk phenotype.[7–9] Despite poor outcomes with surgical aortic valve replacement (SAVR) compared with men, women with severe AS have demonstrated decreased mortality with transcatheter aortic valve replacement (TAVR).[10–13]

Tricuspid regurgitation (TR) is more prevalent among women and is associated with high rates of perioperative mortality.[14] Despite the high prevalence of TR, tricuspid valve (TV) interventions are infrequent and remain associated with comparatively higher rates of morbidity and mortality compared with left-sided valvular interventions among both men and women.[15]

Pregnancy is a susceptible state for women with advanced VHD. Women with severe, stenotic left-sided lesions are at highest risk for HF and poor

Disclosure Statement: The authors have nothing to disclose.
a Division of Cardiology, Harvard Medical School, Massachusetts General Hospital, 55 Fruit Street Yaw 5B, Boston, MA 02114, USA; b Division of Cardiology, Harvard Medical School, Massachusetts General Hospital, 55 Fruit Street Blake 256, Boston, MA 02114, USA
* Corresponding author.
E-mail address: mjwood@mgh.harvard.edu

1551-7136/19/© 2018 Elsevier Inc. All rights reserved.

maternal and neonatal outcomes. The presence of prosthetic valves warrants careful and unique management of anticoagulation in the setting of pregnancy.[16–18]

This review focuses on the sex differences in the epidemiology, diagnosis, treatment, and outcomes of MR, AS, and TR as well as the unique management of VHD in pregnancy.

Mitral Regurgitation

Epidemiology

MR is the leading cause of severe VHD in the United States.[2] MR is a dynamic condition with complex mechanisms and variable disease progression. Although the prevalence of MR is equal among men and women, there are important sex differences in the epidemiology and underlying pathologic condition leading to significant mitral valve (MV) disease.[6]

The leading cause of primary MR is rheumatic heart disease (RHD) in developing countries and degenerative valve disease, predominantly MV prolapse, in the United States.[2] Although MV prolapse is more common in women, women present with lesser degrees of MR compared with men.[19] However, women tend to have increased leaflet thickening and anterior or bileaflet MV prolapse, which can pose unique challenges to MV repair.[3] Women also have a higher prevalence of MV calcification and a predilection for rheumatic MV disease, additional factors challenging their candidacy for routine MV repair.[20]

Women with severe MR undergoing MV surgery typically present at an older age and with more comorbid conditions, including atrial fibrillation, renal insufficiency, and HF.[4] Women's advanced presentation and delay in surgical interventions are likely a combination of patient and provider factors, including women's atypical symptoms, the absence of indexing echocardiographic parameters for BSA for referral to intervention, and the lack of provider familiarity with timing for valvular interventions.[21]

Diagnostic evaluation

Echocardiography remains the gold standard for the evaluation of MR. National guidelines recommend an integrated, multistep approach using qualitative and quantitative echocardiographic parameters for the characterization and grading of MR.[6] Because of the absence of indexed values for size and the prevalence of smaller left ventricular (LV) dimensions among women,[3] the severity of MR is often underestimated by echocardiographic parameters. In a large retrospective cohort of more than 500 men and women who underwent surgical repair for primary MR, preoperatively, women were seldom categorized as having severe LV dilation (13% vs 26%; $P = .0002$) and severe MR (70% vs 81%, $P = .002$) compared with men. However, both parameters were at least as severe in women as in men when indexed for BSA.[20] MRI has recently emerged as an alternative imaging modality with the potential to more accurately assess the severity of MR compared with echocardiography. A multicenter prospective study demonstrated a significant discordance between echocardiography and MRI grading of MR with ventricular volumes demonstrating a stronger correlation with regurgitant volume on MRI compared with commonly used echocardiographic linear dimensions.[22] For patients with discordance between symptoms and echocardiographic severity, particularly among women, follow-up testing using cardiac MRI has a potential role for more accurate quantitation of MR severity.[6] To date, there exist no sex-specific guidelines for the grading of MR or the referral to MV intervention,[6,23,24] exposing women to the risks of underdiagnosis and delayed valvular interventions.

Treatment and outcomes

The decision making regarding the optimal treatment of severe MR is based on a comprehensive assessment of valvular pathologic condition, disease severity, and symptoms. MV surgery is indicated for symptomatic, primary severe MR with LV ejection fraction greater than 30% or in the absence of symptoms with evidence of adverse LV remodeling (LV ejection fraction 30%–60% or LV end systolic dimension $\geq$40 mm).[6,23,24] MV repair has demonstrated superior short- and long-term outcomes over MV replacement among patients with primary MR regardless of age or gender.[25] In contrast, surgical MV repair or replacement has failed to demonstrate any improvement in survival among patients with secondary MR resulting in weaker indications for intervention among this group.[24,26]

Multiple studies have suggested higher mortalities and poor outcomes for women compared with men undergoing isolated MV surgery.[4,27] In general, women are less likely to be referred to surgery, are less likely to receive MV repair, and have worse outcomes associated with MV replacement.[4,5] A retrospective review of the National Inpatient Sample database between 2005 and 2008 demonstrated that women undergo MV repair less often than men (37.9% vs 55.9%, $P<.001$) and more frequently undergo TV surgery and ablation for atrial fibrillation at the time of MV surgery. Although in-hospital mortality was higher among women, this was not significant after adjusting for comorbidities suggestive of women's more advanced clinical presentation.[5] A large comparative study of 47,602 Medicare beneficiaries undergoing isolated MV operations revealed similar findings and additionally demonstrated that, unlike men, MV repair failed to restore life expectancy to that of age- and sex-matched controls among women (**Fig. 1**).[4] Long-term outcomes after MV repair have also shown significant gender disparities with a 10-year survival of 58% in women compared with 72% for men.[27]

New transcatheter options have emerged for patients with severe, primary MR who are not candidates for MV surgery. The transcatheter edge-to-edge MV leaflet coaptation clip (MitraClip (Abott Vascular, Santa Clara, California, USA)) is approved for the treatment of severe, symptomatic degenerative MR in patients at prohibitive risk for MR surgery. In the EVEREST II trial, which randomized patients with at least moderately severe MR to percutaneous repair or conventional surgical repair or replacement, the MitraClip demonstrated superior safety at 30 days but lower efficacy driven by persistent MV dysfunction and residual at least moderate MR (55% vs 73%, $P = .007$) compared with surgery.[28] At 5 years, both techniques were associated with similar degrees of moderate to severe MR without any differences in clinical outcomes.[29] A recent observational registry study found no gender differences in the reduction of MR or New York Heart Association (NYHA) functional class (MR grade ≤2+ in 98.2% of men vs 96.8% of women, $P = .586$, and NYHA class ≤II in 78.3% of men vs 77% of women, $P = .851$) after successful MitraClip placement. There were additionally no gender differences in the incidence of HF or death at 16 months of follow-up.[30] The MitraClip is currently under study for patients with secondary functional MR.[31]

Aortic Stenosis

Epidemiology

AS is the second most common valvular lesion in the United States and is present in about 5% of the population at age 65 with increasing prevalence with advancing age.[2] Degenerative AS is the most common cause of AS secondary to progressive fibrosis and calcification. Although bicuspid aortic valve (AV) disease is the most common type of congenital valvular abnormality, it is more common in men and only accounts for about 1% of all causes of AS in both men and women.[2] Epidemiologic studies have established equal rates of AS among men and women; however, important sex differences exist. Women tend to present later in their disease trajectory with a unique risk profile, including older age, frailty, renal insufficiency, and higher rates of symptomatic HF (NYHA class III–IV), and concomitant moderate to severe MR compared with men.[11] In general, women are also more likely to have smaller annular sizes and LV outflow tract dimensions associated with concentric LV hypertrophy.[7] Women have additionally demonstrated a higher prevalence of paradoxic LF-LG AS, which has been associated with poor outcomes and worse mortality compared with high-gradient AS.[32]

Diagnostic evaluation

Hemodynamically significant AS is defined as a peak aortic jet velocity ≥4 m/s, a mean transvalvular aortic gradient ≥40 mm Hg, and/or an AV area less than 1.0 cm^2.[23] In contrast to MR, echocardiographic guidelines for the diagnosis of AS allow for indexed values for BSA (AV area <0.6 cm^2/m^2), an important distinction for women.[23] A proportion of men and women with AS has a small AV area (≤1.0 cm^2) but low LV outflow velocities and mean gradients indicative of LF (stroke volume index <35 mL/m^2), LG (mean gradient <40 mm Hg) AS.[7] In 5% to 10% of patients, this physiology is caused by depressed LV systolic function. In about 10% to 25% of patients and more commonly among women, a small, restrictive LV cavity results in "paradoxic" underestimation of the severity of

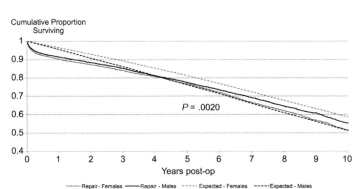

Fig. 1. Ten-year survival for men versus women undergoing MV repair from 2000 to 2009 compared with expected survival in the US population matched for age and sex. (*From* Vassileva CM, McNeely C, Mishkel G, et al. Gender differences in long-term survival of Medicare beneficiaries undergoing mitral valve operations. Ann Thorac Surg 2013;96(4):1371; with permission.)

the AS (paradoxic LF-LG AS) despite preserved LV systolic function.[7]

Considering the technical limitations of echocardiography, recent research has focused on the utility of multidetector computed tomography (MDCT) to improve both diagnostic and prognostic accuracy of patients with severe AS. The degree of AV calcium load by MDCT has been well correlated with the echocardiographic severity of AS.[33] Women have a lower total AV calcium load compared with men for any level of AS severity even after adjustment for BSA.[33–35] Considering these differences, gender-specific calcium scores have been defined (AV calcium ≥1275 arbitrary units [AU] women, ≥2065 AU men) for the diagnosis of AS. Despite lower AV calcium, women have more significant progression of AV calcium over 3 years of follow-up.[9] MDCT has additionally shown efficacy in the identification of calcific severe AS with discordant echocardiographic findings highlighting its unique role in the diagnosis of complex, indeterminate AS cases.[34] The use of MDCT has not been incorporated into the American Heart Association/American College of Cardiology (AHA/ACC) guidelines, representing the need for additional research in this area.[23,24]

Treatment and outcomes

Severe, symptomatic AS carries a poor prognosis without intervention with a 50% rate of mortality at 1 to 2 years.[8] AV replacement carries an AHA/ACC class I recommendation for symptomatic hemodynamically significant AS, severe AS with depressed LV systolic function (<50%), or at least moderate AS in the setting of other cardiac surgery even in the absence of symptoms.[23] Women with severe, symptomatic AS and a class I indication for SAVR are less frequently referred for SAVR (19% lower relative rate, P = .03) compared with men.[36] These results highlight the gender bias that results from the historically higher surgical and in-hospital mortality among women secondary to smaller annular sizes and higher risk of patient-prosthesis mismatch.[37] However, with the emerging role of TAVR, women now account for 50% of patients undergoing TAVR in the United States.[10,13]

Multiple randomized, multicenter clinical trials have now demonstrated both the efficacy and the safety of TAVR in patients with severe, symptomatic AS as an alternative for patients at prohibitive, high, and intermediate risk for SAVR.[38–40] The PARTNER (Placement of Aortic Transcatheter Valve) trial first established the superiority of balloon-expandable TAVR (Edwards Lifesciences, Irvine, CA, USA) compared with medical management by demonstrating a significant reduction in

1-year all-cause mortality among patients with severe AS at prohibitive risk for SAVR (30.7% vs 57.7% [hazard ratio, HR: 0.55; 95% confidence interval, CI: 0.40–0.74]; P<.001)[39] with follow-up PARTNER trials establishing noninferiority of TAVR to SAVR among high-risk and intermediate groups with similar long-term outcomes and improved safety profile at 2 to 5 years of follow-up.[38,40] Similar results have been achieved with TAVR using a different platform with a self-expanding valve Core Valve (Medtronic Inc., Minneapolis, MN, USA).[41,42]

Contrary to SAVR, multiple studies have shown improved survival after TAVR (compared with SAVR) in women, a finding that has not been replicated in men.[11,12,37] A secondary analysis of the PARTNER trials demonstrated that despite a higher incidence of vascular complications and major bleeding among women at 1 year, all-cause mortality (19% vs 25.9%, HR 0.72; CI 0.61–0.85, P<.001) was significantly lower among women compared with men (**Fig. 2**), particularly in women undergoing transfemoral access.[13] Women also showed decreased rates of paravalvular leak (6% vs 14.3%, P<.001) hypothesized to be in part due to less AV calcifications, a well-known risk factor for paravalvular leak.[13] Thus, women may derive greater benefit from TAVR; however, the optimal strategy for women remains undetermined. The WIN-TAVI (Women's International Transcatheter Aortic Valve Implantation) registry is the first all-women single-arm study created to further study the safety and efficacy of TAVR in high- to intermediate-risk women.[10]

TAVR has not been prospectively studied among patients with LF-LG AS[43]; however, LF-LG AS has been shown to carry increased risk of SAVR compared with patients with high-gradient AS.[7] To date, randomized control trials studying the efficacy and safety of TAVR among patients at low surgical risk for SAVR[43] and with severe, asymptomatic AS are ongoing.[44] The AHA/ACC guidelines do not include any specific sex-based recommendations for any surgical or percutaneous intervention for the treatment of severe AS.[24]

Tricuspid Regurgitation

Epidemiology

Severe TR accounts for about 1% to 2% of VHD and is more prevalent among women.[45] More than 90% of severe TR is functional in cause with only a minority of cases caused by trauma, infective endocarditis, or congenital heart disease.[45] Women accounted for 58% of the greater than 45,000 TV surgeries in the United States

A

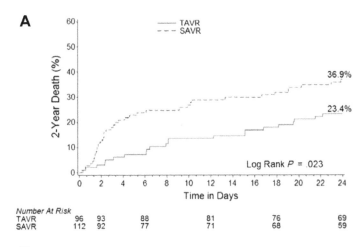

B

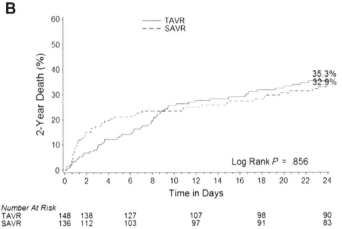

Fig. 2. Differences in all-cause mortality for transfemoral TAVR versus SAVR stratified by sex: (*A*) women, (*B*) men. (*From* Williams M, Kodali SK, Hahn RT, et al. Sex-related differences in outcomes after transcatheter or surgical aortic valve replacement in patients with severe aortic stenosis: insights from the PARTNER Trial (Placement of Aortic Transcatheter Valve). J Am Coll Cardiol 2014;63(15): 1527; with permission.)

performed between 2003 and 2014.[15,46] Untreated severe TR is associated with adverse outcomes; however, surgical intervention is rare, and perioperative mortality is high.[14,47] To date, there exists no AHA/ACC class I indication for surgical intervention among patients with isolated severe TR.[23]

Treatment and outcomes

Treatment of secondary TR focuses on the management of underlying predisposing factors and symptom management. Surgical intervention is only recommended in patients with at least moderate TR undergoing other cardiac surgery.[23,45] Female sex is an independent risk factor for poor perioperative outcomes with combined valve and coronary artery bypass surgery (CABG).[14] The majority (85%) of TV surgeries between 2003 and 2014 occurred at the time of other cardiac surgery, with isolated TV surgery (15%) rarely performed.[15] Isolated TV surgery had high rates in in-hospital mortality (8.8%) among both sexes despite increasing volume of surgical interventions with

significantly higher mortality with TV replacement than TV repair (odds ratio 1.91, 95% CI 1.18–3.09, $P = .009$).[46] In contrast to combined TV surgery at time of CABG surgery, adjusted mortality did not vary by gender in patients undergoing isolated TV surgery.[48] Given the increasing rates of TV interventions and the emerging transcatheter options for severe TR, further research is essential to define perioperative risk factors and optimal surgical timing, particularly among women.[49]

Valvular Heart Disease in Pregnancy

The physiologic and hemodynamic changes associated with pregnancy pose a unique challenge to patients with VHD. Pregnancy is associated with a moderate increase in heart rate and plasma blood volume and a decrease in systemic vascular resistance leading to 30% to 50% increase in cardiac output. Because of these physiologic changes, women with left-sided stenotic lesions are at highest risk for development of symptomatic HF and adverse cardiovascular complications during

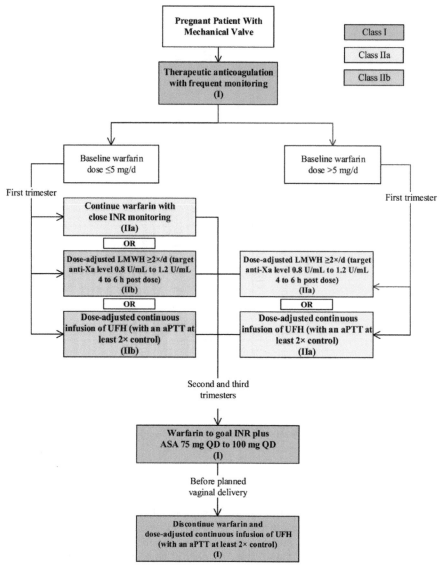

Fig. 3. Anticoagulation of pregnant patients with mechanical valves. aPTT, activated partial thromboplastin time; ASA, acetylsalicylic acid; INR, international normalized ratio; LMWH, low-molecular-weight heparin; QD, daily; UFH, unfractionated heparin. (*From* Nishimura RA, Otto CM, Bonow RO, et al. 2014 AHA/ACC guideline for the management of patients with valvular heart disease: a report of the American College of Cardiology/American Heart Association Task Force on Practice Guidelines. J Thorac Cardiovasc Surg 2014;148(1):2470; with permission.)

pregnancy.[16,17] All women with suspected or diagnosed VHD should undergo preconception planning by a multidisciplinary team consisting of a maternal-fetal specialist and a cardiologist specialized in the care of women through pregnancy.[23]

Aortic stenosis in pregnancy

AS in pregnancy is most often secondary to congenital bicuspid AV stenosis or acquired RHD. Given the association between bicuspid AV and aortic pathologic conditions, dedicated aortic

imaging is recommended before conception.[50] Severe, symptomatic AS and severe aortic dilatation (>50 mm associated with a bicuspid AV) are contraindications to pregnancy given the high risk for adverse maternal and fetal outcomes.[23,50] Although surgical intervention during pregnancy is possible for refractory HF or arrhythmias associated with severe AS, it is associated with 6% maternal and 30% fetal mortalities and should be carefully considered.[18] For high-risk pregnant women with severe AS, balloon valvuloplasty can be used as a bridge to postpartum surgical intervention.[23,50]

Mitral stenosis in pregnancy

Among women of child-bearing age, RHD remains the primary cause of mitral stenosis (MS) in the developing world as well as in the United States. Severe MS is a contraindication to pregnancy and is defined on echocardiography by an MV area of less than 1.5 cm^2 and a diastolic pressure half time greater than 150 milliseconds.[23] Pregnant women with severe MS can become symptomatic due to a decrease in diastolic filling time and resultant increase in left atrial and pulmonary pressures associated with physiologic increases in heart rate in pregnancy. Symptomatic women with refractory HF may require balloon valvulotomy as a bridge to MV replacement post partum.[50]

Prosthetic heart valves in pregnancy

Prosthetic heart valves in pregnant women are associated with a significant increase in maternal and neonatal morbidity. In general, emergent valve replacement for severe VHD is deferred during pregnancy and only considered in the setting of refractory HF or arrhythmias. Existent prosthetic heart valves require meticulous and thoughtful management of anticoagulation during pregnancy. All pregnant women with bioprosthetic heart valves should be treated with low-dose aspirin in the second and third trimesters of pregnancy for the prevention of valve thrombosis. Bioprosthetic heart valves do not require anticoagulation except 3 to 6 months after surgical implantation and in the presence of other thromboembolic risk factors.[23,50] In contrast, women with mechanical heart valves require therapeutic anticoagulation throughout pregnancy. Warfarin is the most effective anticoagulant in the prevention of adverse maternal outcomes, specifically valve thrombosis; however, it has teratogenic effects in the first trimester at doses greater than 5 mg per day and carries a dose-dependent risk of fetal anomalies and pregnancy loss.[51] In contrast, weight-adjusted low-molecular-weight heparin with meticulous anti-Xa level monitoring has proven to be safe and efficacious throughout pregnancy with lower risks of adverse fetal outcomes but higher risk of maternal valve thrombosis.[23,50,51] The current ACC/AHA guidelines recommend the use of warfarin or heparin analogues in the first trimester followed by warfarin therapy for the remainder of the pregnancy (**Fig. 3**). Given the risk-benefit profile of different agents, women should be extensively educated and counseled before making a shared decision on the choice of anticoagulant therapy.

SUMMARY

HF is more prevalent among women, and VHD remains both an important primary contributor and a consequence of progressive HF. Although no gender differences exist in the prevalence of VHD among men and women, important sex differences exist in the diagnosis, treatment, and outcomes of VHD. In addition, the unique physiologic demands of pregnancy are associated with an increased risk of HF in women with VHD. Women have unique valvular pathologic condition, distinct risk factor profiles, and higher prevalence of symptomatic HF, raising the bar for the development of sex-specific recommendations for the tailored diagnosis and treatment of VHD. Future clinical guidelines should address known gender differences to help guide the timely diagnosis and referral to surgical and transcatheter interventions among the growing population of women with VHD. Improving the diagnosis and treatment of advanced VHD among women carries the potential to mitigate the progressive and rapidly increasing prevalence of HF among women.

REFERENCES

1. Benjamin EJ, Virani SS, Callaway CW, et al. Heart disease and stroke statistics-2018 update: a report from the American Heart Association. Circulation 2018;137(12):e67–492.
2. Nkomo VT, Gardin JM, Skelton TN, et al. Burden of valvular heart diseases: a population-based study. Lancet 2006;368(9540):1005–11.
3. Avierinos JF, Inamo J, Grigioni F, et al. Sex differences in morphology and outcomes of mitral valve prolapse. Ann Intern Med 2008;149(11):787–95.
4. Vassileva CM, McNeely C, Mishkel G, et al. Gender differences in long-term survival of Medicare beneficiaries undergoing mitral valve operations. Ann Thorac Surg 2013;96(4):1367–73.
5. Vassileva CM, Stelle LM, Markwell S, et al. Sex differences in procedure selection and outcomes of patients undergoing mitral valve surgery. Heart Surg Forum 2011;14(5):E276–82.
6. O'Gara PT, Grayburn PA, Badhwar V, et al. 2017 ACC expert consensus decision pathway on the management of mitral regurgitation: a report of the American College of Cardiology Task Force on Expert Consensus Decision Pathways. J Am Coll Cardiol 2017;70(19):2421–49.
7. Pibarot P, Dumesnil JG. Low-flow, low-gradient aortic stenosis with normal and depressed left ventricular ejection fraction. J Am Coll Cardiol 2012; 60(19):1845–53.
8. Cramariuc D, Rogge BP, Lønnebakken MT, et al. Sex differences in cardiovascular outcome during

progression of aortic valve stenosis. Heart 2015; 101(3):209–14.

9. Nguyen V, Mathieu T, Melissopoulou M, et al. Sex differences in the progression of aortic stenosis and prognostic implication: the COFRASA-GENERAC Study. JACC Cardiovasc Imaging 2016;9(4):499–501.

10. Chieffo A, Petronio AS, Mehilli J, et al. Acute and 30-day outcomes in women after TAVR: results from the WIN-TAVI (Women's INternational Transcatheter Aortic Valve Implantation) Real-World Registry. JACC Cardiovasc Interv 2016;9(15):1589–600.

11. Chandrasekhar J, Dangas G, Yu J, et al. Sex-based differences in outcomes with transcatheter aortic valve therapy: TVT registry from 2011 to 2014. J Am Coll Cardiol 2016;68(25):2733–44.

12. Williams M, Kodali SK, Hahn RT, et al. Sex-related differences in outcomes after transcatheter or surgical aortic valve replacement in patients with severe aortic stenosis: insights from the PARTNER Trial (Placement of Aortic Transcatheter Valve). J Am Coll Cardiol 2014;63(15):1522–8.

13. Kodali S, Williams MR, Doshi D, et al. Sex-specific differences at presentation and outcomes among patients undergoing transcatheter aortic valve replacement: a cohort study. Ann Intern Med 2016; 164(6):377–84.

14. Ibrahim MF, Paparella D, Ivanov J, et al. Gender-related differences in morbidity and mortality during combined valve and coronary surgery. J Thorac Cardiovasc Surg 2003;126(4):959–64.

15. Zack CJ, Fender EA, Chandrashekar P, et al. National trends and outcomes in isolated tricuspid valve surgery. J Am Coll Cardiol 2017;70(24): 2953–60.

16. Sanghavi M, Rutherford JD. Cardiovascular physiology of pregnancy. Circulation 2014;130(12): 1003–8.

17. Hameed A, Karaalp IS, Tummala PP, et al. The effect of valvular heart disease on maternal and fetal outcome of pregnancy. J Am Coll Cardiol 2001; 37(3):893–9.

18. Weiss BM, von Segesser LK, Alon E, et al. Outcome of cardiovascular surgery and pregnancy: a systematic review of the period 1984-1996. Am J Obstet Gynecol 1998;179(6 Pt 1):1643–53.

19. Avierinos JF, Gersh BJ, Melton LJ 3rd, et al. Natural history of asymptomatic mitral valve prolapse in the community. Circulation 2002;106(11):1355–61.

20. Mantovani F, Clavel MA, Michelena HI, et al. Comprehensive imaging in women with organic mitral regurgitation: implications for clinical outcome. JACC Cardiovasc Imaging 2016;9(4):388–96.

21. Wang A, Grayburn P, Foster JA, et al. Practice gaps in the care of mitral valve regurgitation: insights from the American College of Cardiology mitral regurgitation gap analysis and advisory panel. Am Heart J 2016;172:70–9.

22. Uretsky S, Gillam L, Lang R, et al. Discordance between echocardiography and MRI in the assessment of mitral regurgitation severity: a prospective multicenter trial. J Am Coll Cardiol 2015;65(11): 1078–88.

23. Nishimura RA, Otto CM, Bonow RO, et al. 2014 AHA/ACC guideline for the management of patients with valvular heart disease: a report of the American College of Cardiology/American Heart Association Task Force on Practice Guidelines. J Thorac Cardiovasc Surg 2014;148(1):e1–132.

24. Nishimura RA, Otto CM, Bonow RO, et al. 2017 AHA/ACC focused update of the 2014 AHA/ACC guideline for the management of patients with valvular heart disease: a report of the American College of Cardiology/American Heart Association Task Force on Clinical Practice Guidelines. Circulation 2017; 135(25):e1159–95.

25. Gillinov AM, Blackstone EH, Nowicki ER, et al. Valve repair versus valve replacement for degenerative mitral valve disease. J Thorac Cardiovasc Surg 2008;135(4):885–93, 893.e1-2.

26. Goldstein D, Moskowitz AJ, Gelijns AC, et al. Two-year outcomes of surgical treatment of severe ischemic mitral regurgitation. N Engl J Med 2016; 374(4):344–53.

27. Seeburger J, Eifert S, Pfannmuller B, et al. Gender differences in mitral valve surgery. Thorac Cardiovasc Surg 2013;61(1):42–6.

28. Feldman T, Foster E, Glower DD, et al. Percutaneous repair or surgery for mitral regurgitation. N Engl J Med 2011;364(15):1395–406.

29. Feldman T, Kar S, Elmariah S, et al. Randomized comparison of percutaneous repair and surgery for mitral regurgitation: 5-year results of EVEREST II. J Am Coll Cardiol 2015;66(25):2844–54.

30. Estevez-Loureiro R, Settergren M, Winter R, et al. Effect of gender on results of percutaneous edge-to-edge mitral valve repair with MitraClip system. Am J Cardiol 2015;116(2):275–9.

31. Goldstein NE, Lampert R, Bradley E, et al. Management of implantable cardioverter defibrillators in end-of-life care. Ann Intern Med 2004;141(11):835–8.

32. Saeed S, Senior R, Chahal NS, et al. Lower trans-aortic flow rate is associated with increased mortality in aortic valve stenosis. JACC Cardiovasc Imaging 2017;10(8):912–20.

33. Cueff C, Serfaty JM, Cimadevilla C, et al. Measurement of aortic valve calcification using multislice computed tomography: correlation with haemodynamic severity of aortic stenosis and clinical implication for patients with low ejection fraction. Heart 2011;97(9):721–6.

34. Clavel MA, Messika-Zeitoun D, Pibarot P, et al. The complex nature of discordant severe calcified aortic valve disease grading: new insights from combined Doppler echocardiographic and

computed tomographic study. J Am Coll Cardiol 2013;62(24):2329–38.

35. Clavel MA, Pibarot P, Messika-Zeitoun D, et al. Impact of aortic valve calcification, as measured by MDCT, on survival in patients with aortic stenosis: results of an international registry study. J Am Coll Cardiol 2014;64(12):1202–13.

36. Hartzell M, Malhotra R, Yared K, et al. Effect of gender on treatment and outcomes in severe aortic stenosis. Am J Cardiol 2011;107(11):1681–6.

37. Chaker Z, Badhwar V, Alqahtani F, et al. Sex differences in the utilization and outcomes of surgical aortic valve replacement for severe aortic stenosis. J Am Heart Assoc 2017;6(9) [pii:e006370].

38. Mack MJ, Leon MB, Smith CR, et al. 5-year outcomes of transcatheter aortic valve replacement or surgical aortic valve replacement for high surgical risk patients with aortic stenosis (PARTNER 1): a randomised controlled trial. Lancet 2015;385(9986): 2477–84.

39. Leon MB, Smith CR, Mack M, et al. Transcatheter aortic-valve implantation for aortic stenosis in patients who cannot undergo surgery. N Engl J Med 2010;363(17):1597–607.

40. Leon MB, Smith CR, Mack MJ, et al. Transcatheter or surgical aortic-valve replacement in intermediate-risk patients. N Engl J Med 2016;374(17):1609–20.

41. Adams DH, Popma JJ, Reardon MJ, et al. Transcatheter aortic-valve replacement with a self-expanding prosthesis. N Engl J Med 2014;370(19): 1790–8.

42. Reardon MJ, Van Mieghem NM, Popma JJ, et al. Surgical or transcatheter aortic-valve replacement in intermediate-risk patients. N Engl J Med 2017; 376(14):1321–31.

43. Medtronic C. Medtronic transcatheter aortic valve replacement in low risk patients. 2018. Available at:

https://ClinicalTrials.gov/show/NCT02701283. Accessed February 5, 2018.

44. Edwards L. Evaluation of transcatheter aortic valve replacement compared to surveillance for patients with asymptomatic severe aortic stenosis. 2021. Available at: https://ClinicalTrials.gov/show/NCT03042104. Accessed February 5, 2018.

45. Arsalan M, Walther T, Smith RL 2nd, et al. Tricuspid regurgitation diagnosis and treatment. Eur Heart J 2017;38(9):634–8.

46. Alqahtani F, Berzingi CO, Aljohani S, et al. Contemporary trends in the use and outcomes of surgical treatment of tricuspid regurgitation. J Am Heart Assoc 2017;6(12) [pii:e007597].

47. Topilsky Y, Nkomo VT, Vatury O, et al. Clinical outcome of isolated tricuspid regurgitation. JACC Cardiovasc Imaging 2014;7(12):1185–94.

48. Chandrashekar P, Fender EA, Zack CJ, et al. Sex-stratified analysis of national trends and outcomes in isolated tricuspid valve surgery. Open Heart 2018;5(1):e000719.

49. Taramasso M, Hahn RT, Alessandrini H, et al. The International Multicenter TriValve Registry: which patients are undergoing transcatheter tricuspid repair? JACC Cardiovasc Interv 2017;10(19): 1982–90.

50. Regitz-Zagrosek V, Blomstrom Lundqvist C, Borghi C, et al. ESC guidelines on the management of cardiovascular diseases during pregnancy: the Task Force on the Management of Cardiovascular Diseases during Pregnancy of the European Society of Cardiology (ESC). Eur Heart J 2011;32(24):3147–97.

51. Steinberg ZL, Dominguez-Islas CP, Otto CM, et al. Maternal and fetal outcomes of anticoagulation in pregnant women with mechanical heart valves. J Am Coll Cardiol 2017;69(22):2681–91.

Heart Failure in Women with Congenital Heart Disease

Elisa A. Bradley, MD[a],*, Anita Saraf, MD, PhD[b], Wendy Book, MD[b]

KEYWORDS

- Adult congenital heart disease • Heart failure • Women • Pregnancy

KEY POINTS

- There are limited data on outcomes in women with adult congenital heart disease (ACHD) and heart failure (HF).
- HF is the leading cause of morbidity and mortality in ACHD (women and men).
- The ACHD-HF patient should be evaluated by an ACHD specialist with emphasis on assessing for residual or late ACHD-related complications and correction of these defects if present.
- Management of women with ACHD requires a specialized care team with experience in ACHD.

INTRODUCTION: SCOPE OF THE PROBLEM

Congenital heart disease (CHD) is often thought of as exclusive to children. However, there are now more survivors of adult CHD (ACHD) than there are children with CHD.[1] Recent data derived from Canada and prospectively applied to the US population estimate that there are 1.4 million adults (670,000 men, 775,000 women) living with CHD.[2] Importantly, there are a growing number of patients surviving to adulthood with severely complex CHD.[1,3] This population is at high risk of developing late cardiovascular (CV) complications such as arrhythmia and heart failure (HF).[4–6] In fact, this problem is of such importance that the National Heart Lung and Blood Institute issued a call to action specifically to address the future need for research dedicated to ACHD.[7]

Unlike in the general population, HF is commonly seen in children and young adults with CHD. HF is among the most common late-stage and end-stage complications in moderate and severely complex CHD, accounting for 20% of US hospitalizations in 2007 in the ACHD population.[8] It is also a leading cause of death (27%) after pediatric surgery and/or transplant.[9,10] HF is the cause of death in approximately 28% of hospitalized adults with CHD.[5] Recent data from Spain have shown that women with CHD have worse age-adjusted relative survival (hazard ratio [HR] 1.25, $P = .046$) with HF being the most common reason for death (37% deaths caused by HF).[11] Prior studies have concluded that this is not associated with a history of pregnancy.[12] These data support the need to better understand HF in women with ACHD.

HEART FAILURE IN CONGENITAL HEART DISEASE: A DIFFERENT DISEASE?

In CHD, numerous cardiac defects have a gender-based predilection; defects involving cardiac inflow have a higher incidence in women and outflow tract defects are more common in men.[13] Consequently, women have a higher prevalence of patent ductus arteriosus, Ebstein

Disclosures: All authors have no disclosures related to this project.
[a] Department of Internal Medicine, Division of Cardiovascular Medicine, Dorothy Davis Heart and Lung Research Institute, The Ohio State University, 473 W 12th Avenue Suite 200, Columbus, OH 43210, USA;
[b] Department of Internal Medicine, Division of Cardiovascular Medicine, Emory University, Atlanta, GA, USA
* Corresponding author. 473 West 12th Avenue, DHLRI Suite 200, Columbus, OH 43210.
E-mail address: elisa.bradley@osumc.edu

1551-7136/19/© 2018 Elsevier Inc. All rights reserved.

anomaly, truncus arteriosus, atrioventricular septal defect (AVSD), and tetralogy of Fallot (TOF),[14] which may contribute to differences in the onset and presentation of HF. In the Danish congenital corvitia (CONCOR),[15] a disproportionately higher number of patients who died from HF had an congenitally corrected transposition of the great arteries (CCTGA) or TOF, although gender-based outcomes were not evaluated. Furthermore, the European Heart Survey on CHD found that women were more likely to have limitations due to worse New York Heart Association (NYHA) functional class. To date, there is no clear idea about how CHD-related HF is different in women.

Broadly, ACHD-HF is multifactorial and can result from congenital dysregulation of myocardial architecture, valvular abnormalities, residual obstructive lesions, shunts, and/or arrhythmia. Clinically, the presentation of HF in CHD varies based on anatomy and prior procedures. **Table 1** categorizes some of the more common ACHD-HF phenotypes based on clinical presentation and underlying anatomy.

Pressure Overload Versus Volume Overload

Pressure overload ACHD-HF describes a phenotype that can result from obstruction of either the systemic or pulmonic outflow tract. When obstruction occurs on the systemic side, patients will often present with traditional signs and symptoms of HF, such as reduced exercise tolerance, dyspnea, paroxysmal nocturnal dyspnea, and orthopnea. In the ACHD-HF patient, the phenotype extends beyond that of someone with acquired valve disease, such as aortic stenosis. For example, although patients with coarctation have excellent survival postrepair, more than 10% to 25% of late deaths are due to HF.[16] This has been attributed to abnormal ventricular remodeling, hypertrophy, and diastolic dysfunction.[17] Pressure overload that occurs on the pulmonic ventricular side is often well-tolerated until late, when the patient presents with right HF. Examples of defects causing subpulmonic ventricular pressure overload include TOF and pulmonic stenosis.

Volume overload can also affect either the left-sided or right-sided ventricle. Some common CHD diagnoses that can lead to volume overload of the right ventricle (RV) include pulmonic insufficiency (eg, repaired TOF) and AVSD. Left-sided ventricular volume overload may be caused by conditions such as unrepaired patent ductus AVSD or significant aortic insufficiency.

ACHD-HF becomes complex if patients with a morphologic RV in the systemic ventricular position are considered. The normal RV lacks a middle layer of circular fibers that are integral to radial pumping; however, when subject to pressure overload, such as in dextrotransposition of the great arteries (DTGA) with an atrial switch or congenitally corrected transposition of the great arteries (CCTGA), a middle circular layer can form as a compensatory mechanism. The resultant RV pressure overload can then induce myocardial ischemia and diastolic dysfunction, resulting in HF. In patients with this type of anatomy, premature morbidity and mortality from HF is common.[18]

Complex Congenital Heart Disease

In complex CHD, other factors may modify presentation and risk, such as associated cyanosis or coronary abnormalities.[19,20] Conduction abnormalities, need for pacing, and dysrhythmias are common comorbid conditions in CHD patients, and frequently account for worsening HF symptoms. In CHD patients with prior arrhythmia, there is a 4-fold increase in the incidence of HF.[21] Atrial arrhythmias are more common than ventricular arrhythmias and occur in 15.1% of ACHD patients.[22,23] With a systemic RV (single-ventricle or dual chamber physiologies), 82% of symptomatic and 53% of asymptomatic patients have a documented sustained arrhythmia (>30 minutes).[18] Although there are limited data in women, HF, arrhythmia, stroke, and death are more common in right-sided CHD. Given that these conditions are more prevalent in women, they may be more affected by HF than age-matched men with CHD.[24]

Patients with single-ventricle physiology typically undergo the Fontan operation within the first decade of life. The single ventricle pumps to the systemic circulation and the cavae return directly to the pulmonary arteries, resulting in passive pulmonary blood flow. Failure of the Fontan circuit can occur and is described as 1 of 4 phenotypes[25]: (1) systolic failure, (2) diastolic failure, (3) Fontan failure with normal heart pressures (eg, portal hypertension), and (4) lymphatic abnormalities (protein-losing enteropathy and plastic bronchitis).

WOMEN VERSUS MEN

Very few studies examine gender-specific differences in CHD outcomes, let alone in the context of HF. Oliver and colleagues[11] examined 3311 ACHD subjects at a single center in Spain over 25 years. They found a mortality rate of 10% and showed that women have significantly worse age-adjusted survival compared with men (HR 1.25). Furthermore, HF contributed to death in 43% of women (HF-mediated mortality in men: 30%) and was the leading cause of mortality.

Table 1
Broad phenotypes of adult congenital heart disease–heart failure

ACHD-HF Category	Characteristics	Common CHD Presentation
Pressure overload	• Systemic ventricle (left-sided) HF symptoms: dyspnea, ↓ exercise tolerance, PND • Pulmonic ventricle (right-sided) HF symptoms: usually tolerated until late when symptoms mimic pulmonic ventricular volume overload • Ventricular hypertrophy, laterally displaced PMI • In late stages, dilated and dysfunctional ventricle	• Congenital AS • CoA or interrupted arch • Congenital MS • Shone complex • Subvalvular or supravalvular AS
Volume overload	• Variable presentation • Pulmonic ventricle: peripheral venous congestion, abdominal distention, ↓ appetite, hepatomegaly • Systemic ventricle: Dilatation of the ventricle, pulmonary congestion, dyspnea, ↓ exercise tolerance, PND	• Pulmonic insufficiency (rTOF) • Ebstein with TR • CCTGA with TR • Unrepaired shunt
Systemic RV dysfunction	• Presentation mimics traditional left-sided HF symptoms with: dyspnea, ↓ exercise tolerance, PND • In the case of systemic RV, hypertrophy occurs first followed by dilatation and failure late	• DTGA after atrial switch procedure • CCTGA

Single ventricle and Fontan failure	• In single-ventricle disease, hypertrophy may or may not occur but dilatation eventually ensues followed by left-sided HF symptoms.
	• 4 subtypes[25]:
	  FFrEF: ↓EF, ↑EDP, CO normal, ↑SVR
	  FFpEF: normal EF, ↑ EDP, CO normal, ↑ SVR
	  FFnH: normal EF, EDP, CO, low or normal SVR
	  FFLA: normal EF, EDP, CO, low or normal SVR
	• Presentation varies depending on underlying cause but commonly characterized by exercise intolerance, edema, PLE, refractory ascites, and/or pleural effusions
		• Any single-ventricle condition: TA, DORV, DILV, HLHS, AVSD, mitral atresia, rarely Ebstein

Abbreviations: AS, aortic stenosis; CCTGA, congenitally corrected transposition of the great arteries; CoA, coarctation of the aorta; DILV, double-inlet left ventricle; DORV, double-outlet right ventricle; DTGA, dextrotransposition of the great arteries; FFLA, Fontan failure with lymphatic abnormalities; FFnH, Fontan failure with normal heart; FFpEF, Fontan failure with preserved ejection fraction; FFrEF, Fontan failure with reduced ejection fraction; HLHS, hypoplastic left heart syndrome; MS, mitral stenosis; PLE, protein-losing enteropathy; PMI, point of maximal impulse; PND, paroxysmal nocturnal dyspnea; rTOF, repaired TOF; TA, tricuspid atresia; TR, tricuspid regurgitation.

Although there were no associations that explained the higher mortality in women, the investigators suggested that the higher incidence of pulmonary arterial hypertension (PAH) and pregnancy may contribute to this finding. The Danish CONCOR national registry, which followed 7414 participants over 35 years, may support this hypothesis because PAH was found more commonly in women (33% of the female cohort).[26]

EVALUATION OF HEART FAILURE IN CONGENITAL HEART DISEASE

In adults with CHD it is imperative to recognize and understand both underlying anatomy and previous surgical or percutaneous interventions. HF can occur from primary cardiac dysfunction, hemodynamic compromise from a new or progressive lesion, dysrhythmia, or from extracardiac disease. When evaluating the CHD patient with HF, structural and arrhythmic contributors must first be sought out. Adults with CHD are known to have baseline exercise limitations compared with a non-CHD cohort, making symptom evaluation challenging.[27] Symptoms such as fatigue, dyspnea, and reduced exercise tolerance may not be perceptibly different from baseline. Objective findings may also be skewed in this population because they reflect the underlying anatomic lesion and surgical anatomy. For instance, clinicians lose the ability to use jugular venous pressure as a surrogate of right atrial pressure in complex CHD patients with a Fontan palliation. For a subset of CHD, worsening cyanosis from an intracardiac or extracardiac shunt can be a marker of worsening HF. In many moderate and severely complex CHD patients, arrhythmia accompanies HF and can frequently be the first clinical abnormality to present itself. In all patients with CHD presenting with signs and symptoms of HF, the first step is to evaluate the patient for anatomic sequelae or residua contributing to the presentation.[28] Patients with CHD and HF should be referred to an ACHD specialist for further evaluation and treatment. A reasonable approach to the ACHD-HF patient is outlined in **Fig. 1**.

STANDARD HEART FAILURE THERAPY IN CONGENITAL HEART DISEASE PATIENTS
Medications

After structural and arrhythmic contributors to HF have been addressed, HF therapy mirrors that used in the acquired-HF population. Clinical trials in CHD are limited by a small population size with heterogeneous disease and data are extrapolated from the non-CHD population, with little evidence in CHD groups. For the CHD patient with known left-sided systolic dysfunction and HF symptoms, it is reasonable to initiate guideline-based HF therapies such as have been studied in the non-CHD population.[9,29] The rationale is that beta-blockers and angiotensin-converting enzyme inhibitors (ACEis) reduce the negative effects of neurohormonal activation[16] in patients with left ventricular remodeling,[30] fibrosis,[31] and hypertrophy. Selected HF medications and data on use in ACHD-HF are outlined in **Table 2**.[32–43] Fontan failure is a complicated and multifactorial diagnosis that is unique and best managed at an ACHD center.

Mechanical Circulatory Support and Heart Transplant

In the CHD patient that has received maximal medical therapy or intervention for potential reversible causes of HF, yet has persistent advanced HF symptoms, orthotopic heart transplant (OHT) may be an option for suitable candidates.[44] For select patients, mechanical circulatory support (MCS) may be an option. The data evaluating MCS in the CHD population are sparse, in part because MCS is used in a minority of patients[45] and mortality may be worse in this group.[46]

The use of MCS in the CHD population is limited for many reasons, the most important of which is underlying anatomic considerations. To be more specific, anomalies associated with abnormal cardiac rotation lead to atypical geometry of the outflow tracts and device placement is more challenging; therefore, there is a higher risk. This risk is compounded by prior sternotomies and scar. However, MCS have been used successfully in the case of systemic RV failure that can occur in CCTGA or DTGA after atrial switch operation (Mustard or Senning). In the single-ventricle Fontan patient, mechanical assist in the usual context is not typically helpful because systolic function is frequently normal in the adult population. Instead, HF in this group requires understanding of complex Fontan physiology and, even when it is thought that cavopulmonary assist would be helpful, the unfortunate truth is that there is no such device currently available. This remains an active area of study and MCS use in the CHD population is of intense interest, highlighting the need for further research in this area.[44]

Several groups have examined OHT survival in ACHD and found that, although 1-year survival is worse (early mortality odds ratio 4.18) in the CHD population,[47] conditional survival based on survival to year 1 is significantly better than OHT for other indications.[46,48–53] It has been thought that

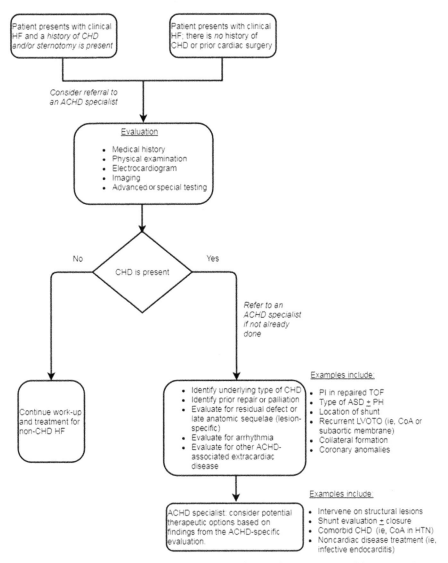

Fig. 1. Evaluation of HF when ACHD may be present. This figure shows a reasonable approach to evaluating a new patient with HF, and in particular highlights how the adult patient with congenital heart disease should be triaged. ACHD, adult congenital heart disease; ASD; atrial septal defect, CHD, congenital heart disease, CoA, Coarctation of the aorta, HF, heart failure, PI, pulmonic insufficiency, HTN: hypertension, LVOTO: left ventricular outflow tract obstruction, PH: pulmonary hypertension, TOF: tetralogy of Fallot.

early survival is compromised in the CHD population due to several factors: technically difficult surgery (repeat sternotomy), longer ischemic time, higher bleeding risk, antibody sensitization, presence of extracardiac disease, and requirement for extracorporeal membrane oxygenation, among others. The improved late survival in conditional 1-year survivors likely relates to the relatively young age, with fewer comorbidities, of ACHD patients undergoing transplant. Data from the United Network of Organ Sharing (UNOS) organization have shown that, although use of MCS has led to reduced wait-list mortality in the non-CHD population, the converse is true in ACHD in which mortality is higher, independent of the type of MCS used.[46] Interestingly, in the same study, women with CHD fared better than men when transplanted. The complexities of OHT in the ACHD population are compounded by the current UNOS listing strategy, which does not adequately take into account the heterogeneity among the CHD population, particularly the experience with MCS and lack of cavopulmonary support. Several investigators have called for more extensive investigation of the ACHD population in the area of transplant medicine.[9,39,44]

Table 2
Standard heart failure medical therapy in congenital heart disease patients

Medication	Selected Data on Use in ACHD-HF
Beta-blockers	• Beneficial with isolated LV systolic dysfunction and with isolated left-sided valvular regurgitation[33,35,36] • Less clear benefit in RV failure • May improve short-term HF symptoms in CHD[32,34]
ACE inhibitors, angiotensin blockers	• No clear benefit has been shown in CHD patients[37–39] • May be beneficial in LV systolic dysfunction
Aldosterone antagonists	• In 3 patients with Fontan physiology, there was remission of PLE with spironolactone[69] • In Fontan patients there was no change in endothelial function or biomarkers when patients were administered spironolactone[43]
Anticoagulation	• Coumadin use has shown good efficacy when anticoagulation is indicated[41] • Caution in patients with cyanosis and erythrocytosis (Hct >55%), low overall plasma volume leads to falsely increased INR[41] • In high-risk patients, antiplatelet therapy has been found to be noninferior to coumadin[41] • Newer direct oral anticoagulants are currently being studied in the ACHD population
Pulmonary arterial vasodilators	• In ES patients, short-term 6-min walk test improved with ERA therapy[40] • In ES, long-term 6-min walk test improved with ERA therapy[42] • Some studies have shown no survival benefit in CHD patients with pulmonary arterial hypertension,[42,70] whereas other studies have shown survival benefit[71]

Abbreviations: ACE, angiotensin converting enzyme; ERA, endothelin receptor antagonist; ES, Eisenmenger syndrome; Hct, hematocrit; LV, left ventricle.

PREGNANCY AND HEART FAILURE IN ADULT CONGENITAL HEART DISEASE

Survival to reproductive years is expected even in the most complex forms of CHD. For women it becomes important to assess the maternal CV risk of pregnancy and labor or delivery. The Canadian Cardiac Disease in Pregnancy[54] and Zwangerschap bij Aangeboren HARtAfwijkingen (ZAHARA)[55] scores are the most widely cited maternal risk stratification tools used in the ACHD patient, along with applying the modified World Health Organization classification of maternal CV risk.[56] Each of these stratification tools identifies that women with ACHD and HF are among the highest risk patients during pregnancy.[54,55] For women with ACHD and HF who undertake pregnancy, there is a substantial risk of further decline in heart function.[57,58] Pregnancy is generally contraindicated in women with significant systemic ventricular dysfunction (ejection fraction <30%) and advanced HF symptoms (NYHA class III or IV); therefore, counseling should include a frank discussion of this risk.[56]

Management of the ACHD patient with HF requires a specialized high-risk team made up of obstetricians with expertise in maternal fetal medicine, congenital cardiologists, cardiac and obstetric anesthesiologists, neonatologists; a tertiary care center where nurses and support staff have experience with these high-risk patients; and availability of advanced MCS and OHT.[28,56,59,60] Medical management involves optimizing HF medications, in particular the discontinuation of agents toxic to the fetus (eg, ACEi, angiotensin receptor blockers, aldosterone antagonists) while titrating nontoxic HF medications (eg, beta blockers, hydralazine, nitrates). Typically, these women have regular follow-up, minimally at each trimester if stable and more frequently in those with symptoms or evidence of early decompensation (**Table 3**).

In most cases, even patients with moderate and severely complex CHD will have a vaginal delivery. Induction may be recommended so that there is more control over labor and delivery. Timing of induction is a decision that should be made in

Table 3
Antepartum congenital heart disease cardiovascular evaluation

	Clinical Evaluation	Diagnostic Testing
First trimester (0–14 wk)	Review cardiac history and recent CV testing History should focus on any underlying CV symptoms (eg, dyspnea, exercise intolerance, palpitations) Review cardiac medications and adjust if necessary Low-risk asymptomatic patients can be followed locally after initial evaluation Moderate and severely complex CHD patients require subsequent follow-up	• Consider echocardiography if there is not a recent evaluation of CV structure and function
Second trimester (14–28 wk)	Detailed history and physical examination focusing on symptoms and any evaluating for any evidence of HF or arrhythmia Moderate-severely complex CHD patients should be discussed with the multidisciplinary specialized care team to formalize labor or delivery and postpartum care plans by the end of this trimester	• Consider echocardiography if volume load could affect underlying physiology • Fetal echocardiography at 18–22 wk to screen for CHD in the fetus[68]
Third trimester (28–42 wk)	Follow-up is similar to the second trimester, with particular focus on discriminating between normal signs and symptoms of late pregnancy and those of worsening CV status Delivery plans are finalized with the multidisciplinary team at this time.	• Directed by patient presentation

concert with the multidisciplinary specialized CV, obstetric, and maternal fetal medicine team. Careful consultation with an anesthesiology team experienced in high-risk obstetric and CV care is required when considering the underlying cardiac anatomy, physiology, and the effect of anesthetic in moderate and severely complex patients. In most cases, it is optimal to pursue a vaginal delivery with adequate analgesia; cesarean section may be recommended but typically is indicated for an obstetric, rather than CV, indication. In some cases it may be recommended that the second stage of labor be assisted (vacuum or forceps-assisted delivery), particularly in women with compromised CV function. In the patient who has an underlying right-to-left shunt, access lines should have air filters to prevent air paradoxic embolism. Intrapartum monitoring will often include telemetry and may require oxygen saturation monitoring, particularly in the patient with a known shunt and/or underlying cyanosis.[56] Women with severely complex CHD may also need invasive hemodynamic monitoring. Particularly, the CHD patient with HF needs to be assessed for the use of peripartum central venous and arterial access for monitoring. These patients may be cared for in an intensive care setting during the intrapartum and immediate postpartum phases. Although there are no cardiac guidelines that support intrapartum antibiotic use for endocarditis prophylaxis, some investigators have suggested it is reasonable in high-risk patients.[56] Postpartum monitoring of the CHD patient with HF or at high risk for HF will require telemetry monitoring at least 24 hours postpartum, as well as careful clinical monitoring for evidence of decompensated HF and development of arrhythmia. Contraception should be addressed before hospital discharge. These patients should be evaluated in the outpatient setting within a few weeks of hospital discharge because the risk for recurrent or worsening HF can occur up to 8 weeks after delivery.[61–68]

REFERENCES

1. Marelli AJ, Ionescu-Ittu R, Mackie AS, et al. Lifetime prevalence of congenital heart disease in the general population from 2000 to 2010. Circulation 2014;130:749–56.

2. Gilboa SM, Devine OJ, Kucik JE, et al. Congenital heart defects in the United States: estimating the magnitude of the affected population in 2010. Circulation 2016;134:101–9.

3. Marelli AJ, Mackie AS, Ionescu-Ittu R, et al. Congenital heart disease in the general population: changing prevalence and age distribution. Circulation 2007;115:163–72.

4. Norozi K, Wessel A, Alpers V, et al. Incidence and risk distribution of heart failure in adolescents and adults with congenital heart disease after cardiac surgery. Am J Cardiol 2006;97:1238–43.

5. Engelings CC, Helm PC, Abdul-Khaliq H, et al. Cause of death in adults with congenital heart disease - An analysis of the German National Register for Congenital Heart Defects. Int J Cardiol 2016; 211:31–6.

6. Kantor PF, Redington AN. Pathophysiology and management of heart failure in repaired congenital heart disease. Heart Fail Clin 2010;6:497–506, ix.

7. Gurvitz M, Burns KM, Brindis R, et al. Emerging research directions in adult congenital heart disease: a report from an NHLBI/ACHA working group. J Am Coll Cardiol 2016;67:1956–64.

8. Opotowsky AR, Siddiqi OK, Webb GD. Trends in hospitalizations for adults with congenital heart disease in the U.S. J Am Coll Cardiol 2009;54: 460–7.

9. Stout KK, Broberg CS, Book WM, et al, American Heart Association Council on Clinical Cardiology, Council on Functional Genomics and Translational Biology, and Council on Cardiovascular Radiology and Imaging. Chronic heart failure in congenital heart disease: a scientific statement from the American Heart Association. Circulation 2016;133: 770–801.

10. Nieminen HP, Jokinen EV, Sairanen HI. Causes of late deaths after pediatric cardiac surgery: a population-based study. J Am Coll Cardiol 2007; 50:1263–71.

11. Oliver JM, Gallego P, Gonzalez AE, et al. Impact of age and sex on survival and causes of death in adults with congenital heart disease. Int J Cardiol 2017;245:119–24.

12. Zomer AC, Ionescu-Ittu R, Vaartjes I, et al. Sex differences in hospital mortality in adults with congenital heart disease: the impact of reproductive health. J Am Coll Cardiol 2013;62:58–67.

13. Engelfriet P, Mulder BJ. Gender differences in adult congenital heart disease. Neth Heart J 2009;17:414–7.

14. Samanek M. Boy:girl ratio in children born with different forms of cardiac malformation: a population-based study. Pediatr Cardiol 1994;15:53–7.

15. Zomer AC, Vaartjes I, Uiterwaal CS, et al. Circumstances of death in adult congenital heart disease. Int J Cardiol 2012;154:168–72.

16. Schrier RW, Abraham WT. Hormones and hemodynamics in heart failure. N Engl J Med 1999;341: 577–85.

17. Krieger EV, Fernandes SM. Heart failure caused by congenital left-sided lesions. Heart Fail Clin 2014; 10:155–65.

18. Piran S, Veldtman G, Siu S, et al. Heart failure and ventricular dysfunction in patients with single or systemic right ventricles. Circulation 2002;105:1189–94.

19. O'Connor WN, Cash JB, Cottrill CM, et al. Ventriculo-coronary connections in hypoplastic left hearts: an autopsy microscopic study. Circulation 1982;66: 1078–86.

20. Baffa JM, Chen SL, Guttenberg ME, et al. Coronary artery abnormalities and right ventricular histology in hypoplastic left heart syndrome. J Am Coll Cardiol 1992;20:350–8.

21. Yang H, Kuijpers JM, de Groot JR, et al. Impact of atrial arrhythmias on outcome in adults with congenital heart disease. Int J Cardiol 2017;248:152–4.

22. Karbassi A, Nair K, Harris L, et al. Atrial tachyarrhythmia in adult congenital heart disease. World J Cardiol 2017;9:496–507.

23. Bouchardy J, Therrien J, Pilote L, et al. Atrial arrhythmias in adults with congenital heart disease. Circulation 2009;120:1679–86.

24. Bernier M, Marelli AJ, Pilote L, et al. Atrial arrhythmias in adult patients with right- versus left-sided congenital heart disease anomalies. Am J Cardiol 2010;106:547–51.

25. Book WM, Gerardin J, Saraf A, et al. Clinical phenotypes of Fontan failure: implications for management. Congenit Heart Dis 2016;11:296–308.

26. Verheugt CL, Uiterwaal CS, van der Velde ET, et al. Gender and outcome in adult congenital heart disease. Circulation 2008;118:26–32.

27. Kempny A, Dimopoulos K, Uebing A, et al. Reference values for exercise limitations among adults with congenital heart disease. Relation to activities of daily life–single centre experience and review of published data. Eur Heart J 2012;33: 1386–96.

28. Silversides CK, Marelli A, Beauchesne L, et al. Canadian Cardiovascular Society 2009 Consensus Conference on the management of adults with

congenital heart disease: executive summary. Can J Cardiol 2010;26:143–50.

29. Book WM, Shaddy RE. Medical therapy in adults with congenital heart disease. Heart Fail Clin 2014; 10:167–78.

30. Kehat I, Molkentin JD. Molecular pathways underlying cardiac remodeling during pathophysiological stimulation. Circulation 2010;122:2727–35.

31. Chapman RE, Spinale FG. Extracellular protease activation and unraveling of the myocardial interstitium: critical steps toward clinical applications. Am J Physiol Heart Circ Physiol 2004;286:H1–10.

32. Doughan AR, McConnell ME, Book WM. Effect of beta blockers (carvedilol or metoprolol XL) in patients with transposition of great arteries and dysfunction of the systemic right ventricle. Am J Cardiol 2007;99:704–6.

33. Ennis DB, Rudd-Barnard GR, Li B, et al. Changes in mitral annular geometry and dynamics with β-blockade in patients with degenerative mitral valve disease. Circ Cardiovasc Imaging 2010;3: 687–93.

34. Farha S, Saygin D, Park MM, et al. Pulmonary arterial hypertension treatment with carvedilol for heart failure: a randomized controlled trial. JCI Insight 2017;2 [pii:95240].

35. Plante E, Lachance D, Champetier S, et al. Benefits of long-term beta-blockade in experimental chronic aortic regurgitation. Am J Physiol Heart Circ Physiol 2008;294:H1888–95.

36. Zendaoui A, Lachance D, Roussel E, et al. Usefulness of carvedilol in the treatment of chronic aortic valve regurgitation. Circ Heart Fail 2011;4:207–13.

37. Anderson RH, Ho SY, Redmann K, et al. The anatomical arrangement of the myocardial cells making up the ventricular mass. Eur J Cardiothorac Surg 2005;28:517–25.

38. Bolger AP, Sharma R, Li W, et al. Neurohormonal activation and the chronic heart failure syndrome in adults with congenital heart disease. Circulation 2002;106:92–9.

39. Budts W, Roos-Hesselink J, Radle-Hurst T, et al. Treatment of heart failure in adult congenital heart disease: a position paper of the Working Group of Grown-Up Congenital Heart Disease and the Heart Failure Association of the European Society of Cardiology. Eur Heart J 2016;37:1419–27.

40. Galie N, Beghetti M, Gatzoulis MA, et al, Bosentan Randomized Trial of Endothelin Antagonist Therapy-5 (BREATHE-5) Investigators. Bosentan therapy in patients with Eisenmenger syndrome: a multicenter, double-blind, randomized, placebo-controlled study. Circulation 2006;114:48–54.

41. Jensen AS, Idorn L, Norager B, et al. Anticoagulation in adults with congenital heart disease: the who, the when and the how? Heart 2015;101: 424–9.

42. Kaya MG, Lam YY, Erer B, et al. Long-term effect of bosentan therapy on cardiac function and symptomatic benefits in adult patients with Eisenmenger syndrome. J Card Fail 2012;18:379–84.

43. Mahle WT, Wang A, Quyyumi AA, et al. Impact of spironolactone on endothelial function in patients with single ventricle heart. Congenit Heart Dis 2009;4:12–6.

44. Ross HJ, Law Y, Book WM, et al. Transplantation and mechanical circulatory support in congenital heart disease: a scientific statement From the American Heart Association. Circulation 2016; 133:802–20.

45. Gelow JM, Song HK, Weiss JB, et al. Organ allocation in adults with congenital heart disease listed for heart transplant: impact of ventricular assist devices. J Heart Lung Transplant 2013;32:1059–64.

46. Davies RR, Russo MJ, Yang J, et al. Listing and transplanting adults with congenital heart disease. Circulation 2011;123:759–67.

47. Singh TP, Almond CS, Semigran MJ, et al. Risk prediction for early in-hospital mortality following heart transplantation in the United States. Circ Heart Fail 2012;5:259–66.

48. Bradley EA, Pinyoluksana KO, Moore-Clingenpeel M, et al. Isolated heart transplant and combined heart-liver transplant in adult congenital heart disease patients: Insights from the united network of organ sharing. Int J Cardiol 2017;228:790–5.

49. Bhama JK, Shulman J, Bermudez CA, et al. Heart transplantation for adults with congenital heart disease: results in the modern era. J Heart Lung Transplant 2013;32:499–504.

50. Chen JM, Davies RR, Mital SR, et al. Trends and outcomes in transplantation for complex congenital heart disease: 1984 to 2004. Ann Thorac Surg 2004;78:1352–61 [discussion: 1352–61].

51. Lamour JM, Kanter KR, Naftel DC, et al. The effect of age, diagnosis, and previous surgery in children and adults undergoing heart transplantation for congenital heart disease. J Am Coll Cardiol 2009; 54:160–5.

52. Lewis M, Ginns J, Schulze C, et al. Outcomes of adult patients with congenital heart disease after heart transplantation: impact of disease type, previous thoracic surgeries, and bystander organ dysfunction. J Card Fail 2016;22:578–82.

53. Simpson KE, Esmaeeli A, Khanna G, et al. Liver cirrhosis in Fontan patients does not affect 1-year post-heart transplant mortality or markers of liver function. J Heart Lung Transplant 2014;33:170–7.

54. Siu SC, Sermer M, Colman JM, et al. Prospective multicenter study of pregnancy outcomes in women with heart disease. Circulation 2001;104:515–21.

55. Drenthen W, Boersma E, Balci A, et al. Predictors of pregnancy complications in women with congenital heart disease. Eur Heart J 2010;31:2124–32.

56. Canobbio MM, Warnes CA, Aboulhosn J, et al, American Heart Association Council on Cardiovascular and Stroke Nursing; Council on Clinical Cardiology; Council on Cardiovascular Disease in the Young; Council on Functional Genomics and Translational Biology; and Council on Quality of Care and Outcomes Research. Management of pregnancy in patients with complex congenital heart disease: a scientific statement for healthcare professionals from the American Heart Association. Circulation 2017;135:e50–87.

57. Bowater SE, Selman TJ, Hudsmith LE, et al. Long-term outcome following pregnancy in women with a systemic right ventricle: is the deterioration due to pregnancy or a consequence of time? Congenit Heart Dis 2013;8:302–7.

58. Guedes A, Mercier LA, Leduc L, et al. Impact of pregnancy on the systemic right ventricle after a Mustard operation for transposition of the great arteries. J Am Coll Cardiol 2004;44:433–7.

59. Regitz-Zagrosek V, Blomstrom Lundqvist C, Borghi C, et al. ESC Guidelines on the management of cardiovascular diseases during pregnancy: the Task Force on the Management of Cardiovascular Diseases during Pregnancy of the European Society of Cardiology (ESC). Eur Heart J 2011;32:3147–97.

60. Whittemore R, Hobbins JC, Engle MA. Pregnancy and its outcome in women with and without surgical treatment of congenital heart disease. Am J Cardiol 1982;50:641–51.

61. Kjeldsen J. Hemodynamic investigations during labour and delivery. Acta Obstet Gynecol Scand Suppl 1979;89:1–252.

62. Robson SC, Dunlop W, Moore M, et al. Combined Doppler and echocardiographic measurement of cardiac output: theory and application in pregnancy. Br J Obstet Gynaecol 1987;94:1014–27.

63. Milne JA, Howie AD, Pack AI. Dyspnoea during normal pregnancy. Br J Obstet Gynaecol 1978;85:260–3.

64. Hirnle L, Lysenko L, Gerber H, et al. Respiratory function in pregnant women. Adv Exp Med Biol 2013;788:153–60.

65. Hendricks CH, Quilligan EJ. Cardiac output during labor. Am J Obstet Gynecol 1956;71:953–72.

66. Robson SC, Dunlop W, Boys RJ, et al. Cardiac output during labour. Br Med J (Clin Res Ed) 1987;295:1169–72.

67. Ueland K, Hansen JM. Maternal cardiovascular dynamics. 3. Labor and delivery under local and caudal analgesia. Am J Obstet Gynecol 1969;103:8–18.

68. Adams JQ, Alexander AM Jr. Alterations in cardiovascular physiology during labor. Obstet Gynecol 1958;12:542–9.

69. Ringel RE, Peddy SB. Effect of high-dose spironolactone on protein-losing enteropathy in patients with Fontan palliation of complex congenital heart disease. Am J Cardiol 2003;91:1031–2. A9.

70. Diller GP, Dimopoulos K, Kaya MG, et al. Long-term safety, tolerability and efficacy of bosentan in adults with pulmonary arterial hypertension associated with congenital heart disease. Heart 2007;93:974–6.

71. Dimopoulos K, Inuzuka R, Goletto S, et al. Improved survival among patients with Eisenmenger syndrome receiving advanced therapy for pulmonary arterial hypertension. Circulation 2010;121:20–5.

Advanced Therapies for Advanced Heart Failure in Women

Marlena V. Habal, MD*, Kelly Axsom, MD,
Maryjane Farr, MD, MSc

KEYWORDS

- Advanced heart failure • Cardiogenic shock • Women • Left ventricular assist device
- Percutaneous mechanical circulatory support

KEY POINTS

- Compared with their male counterparts, women with advanced heart failure and cardiogenic shock are more likely to present with a higher risk profile, older age, more comorbidities, and a higher left ventricular ejection fraction.
- Women are underrepresented in trials of both short-term mechanical circulatory support and durable left ventricular assist device (LVAD).
- Women with acute decompensated heart failure frequently receive less intensive medical and invasive interventions, including short-term mechanical circulatory support from which they derive similar benefit.
- The smaller size of newer generation LVADs has increased the feasibility of offering durable left ventricular support to women.
- Although women are at increased risk of stroke after LVAD, newer devices with a more favorable stroke risk profile may reduce this complication.
- The psychosocial issues surrounding advanced therapies and LVAD present unique challenges among women. Further studies are urgently needed to improve the understanding and appropriate use of durable support.

PART I: INPATIENT MANAGEMENT OF ACUTE DECOMPENSATED HEART FAILURE IN WOMEN

Introduction

Advanced heart failure (HF) is characterized by refractory symptoms, recurrent hospitalizations, and severe impairment in functional capacity.[1–3] Although, overall, men and women are affected in equal numbers, women are consistently underrepresented in clinical trials.[4]

The understanding of the presentation, treatment, and prognosis of hospitalized women with advanced decompensated HF (ADHF) stems predominantly from registry data. In the setting of acute HF, these include the Acute Decompensated Heart Failure National Registry (ADHERE) and the Organized Program to Initiate Lifesaving Treatment in Hospitalized Patients with Heart Failure (OPTIMIZE-HF) study, in which women and men were equally represented (52% women, 48% men).[5,6] In contrast, women made up only

Disclosure: The authors have nothing to disclose.
Department of Medicine, Division of Cardiology, Center for Advanced Cardiac Care, Columbia University Medical Center, 622 West 168th Street PH1273, New York, NY 10032, USA
* Corresponding author.
E-mail address: mh3696@cumc.columbia.edu

Heart Failure Clin 15 (2019) 97–107
https://doi.org/10.1016/j.hfc.2018.08.010
1551-7136/19/© 2018 Elsevier Inc. All rights reserved.

36% of patients in the Should We Emergently Revascularize Occluded Coronaries for Cardiogenic Shock (SHOCK) Registry and 31% in the SHOCK II trial.[7,8] This underrepresentation of women in studies of cardiogenic shock continues in the contemporary era with women making up 21% of patients in the Interagency Registry for Mechanically Assisted Circulatory Support (INTERMACS) registry[9] and less than one-third of patients in studies of percutaneous mechanical support. A summary of these studies is provided in **Table 1**.

Gender Differences in the Presentation and Prognosis of Acute Decompensated Heart Failure and Cardiogenic Shock

Women typically present at an older age, have more comorbidities (eg, hypertension), and a higher left ventricular ejection fraction (LVEF).[5–8] Acutely, both men and women present with symptoms of congestion and/or hypoperfusion in the setting of decompensated HF and cardiogenic shock with a trend toward more congestion (orthopnea and rales) among women.[5,10] From a hemodynamic perspective, women in the SHOCK registry presented with a lower cardiac power index,[7] an established marker of prognosis. In advanced HF, women present similarly to men except for a marginally higher central venous pressure (CVP).[11]

There is some degree of heterogeneity in the literature regarding prognosis. The first consideration relates to differences in cause. In a cohort of participants with chronic HF admitted with ADHF, compared with their male counterparts, women with an ischemic cardiomyopathy had higher all-cause mortality (hazard ratio [HR] 1.95, CI 0.98–3.90, $P = .05$) whereas those with a nonischemic cause had lower all-cause mortality (HR 0.40, 95% CI 0.17–0.96, $P = .01$).[11] The second point to consider, however, is that women tend to present with a higher risk profile given their older age and higher burden of comorbidities. This emphasizes the importance of considering both crude and adjusted outcomes. Indeed, in the setting of ischemia, historical data suggested that women had increased risk for HF and cardiogenic shock with higher mortality.[12–14] However, after adjustment for age, outcomes were similar.[14,15] In the SHOCK registry despite women having a higher baseline risk profile (older age, more diabetes, hypertension, and lower cardiac index), mortality did not differ between men and women among participants who underwent revascularization and those managed conservatively.[7] Similarly, in ADHERE and OPTIMIZE-HF, there were no significant gender-related differences in

risk-adjusted mortality. Recent studies of contemporary mechanical circulatory support (MCS) have reported similar findings, although women continue to be underrepresented.[16,17]

Inpatient Therapies for Advanced Acute Decompensated Heart Failure in Women

When considering inpatient management, 3 essential questions emerge. First, are women offered the same therapies as their male counterparts? Second, are there gender differences in the response to these therapies? Finally, what are the outcomes of women with ADHF?

Continuing a common theme, women remain underrepresented in trials of inpatient medical management for ADHF and cardiogenic shock.[18–20] Although some studies provided subgroup analyses to assess for gender-related differences, others have failed to do so, and the underrepresentation of women further limits generalizability. However, registry data have shed light on the similarities and differences in the utilization and response to inpatient medical therapies for ADHF.

Diuretic and Vasoactive Therapies

In ADHERE, intravenous diuretics were commonly used among both women and men (87% vs 89%, respectively). However, mean weight change was significantly lower for women compared with men both overall (−2.5 ± 4.5 kg vs –3.4 ± 5.0 kg) and in the subgroup with preserved LVEF. Similarly, in the OPTIMIZE-HF registry, less weight loss was achieved (−1.4 kg [−4.0–0 kg] vs −2.3 kg [−5.0–0 kg], $P <.001$). This may be due to lower dosages and/or fewer dose increases.[10]

Intravenous vasoactive therapies are less frequently used for women. In ADHERE, 24% of women compared with 31% of men were treated with vasoactive agents ($P <.0001$). Moreover, the mean time to therapy was longer (24.5 ± 56.6 h vs 22.9 ± 50.8 h, $P = .009$) and the duration of therapy was shorter (3.2 ± 4.4 vs 4.1 ± 7.2 days, $P <.0001$). Similar discrepancies in the use of inotropic therapies have been reported in the large EuroHeart Failure Survey (EHFS) II, suggesting that this less aggressive treatment of women is not unique to North America.[21]

These findings raise the question of whether there are differences in tolerability and hemodynamic response to inpatient therapies between men and women. This was eloquently answered in a retrospective review of 278 participants (19% women) with New York Heart Association (NYHA) class III and IV chronic systolic HF who were admitted with ADHF.[11] All participants received a pulmonary artery catheter. At baseline,

Table 1
Representation of women in registries of cardiogenic shock and acute decompensated heart failure

	Cardiogenic Shock			ADHF	
	SHOCK Registry[7,a]	IABP-SHOCK II[8]	cVAD Registry[16]	ADHERE[6]	PROTECT[10]
Women (%)	36.4%	31%	27.2%	52%	33%
Year	1993–1997	2009–2012	2007–2013	2001–2004	2007–2009
Selected baseline differences (women vs men)	Older ($71.4 + 11.1$ vs $66.8 + 12.3$ y) Less likely to have had a prior MI (32.0% vs 44.7%) Other comorbidities: • HTN (62.1% vs 45.6%) • Diabetes (40.8% vs 28.3%) Less likely to be a smoker (40.7% vs 57.5%)	Older (74 vs 68 y) Less likely to have had a prior MI (16% vs 25%) More comorbidities: • HTN (76% vs 66%) • Diabetes (40% vs 29%) Less likely to be a smoker (25% vs 39%)	Older (71.0 ± 12.8 vs 63.8 ± 13.0 y) No significant difference in prior MI (32.7% vs 34.8%) Trend toward more comorbidities: • HTN (79.6% vs 69.4%) • Diabetes (54.2% vs 41.1%) Less likely to be a smoker (25.5% vs 53.4%)	Older (74.5 ± 14 vs 70.1 ± 14 y) Less likely to have an ischemic cause (19% vs 32%) More HTN and thyroid disease Less hyperlipidemia, renal insufficiency, and smoking	Older (73 ± 11 vs 69 ± 12 y) Less likely to have an ischemic cause (66% vs 72%) More HTN and diabetes Less smoking and COPD
Presentation	No significant differences: • MI location • Time from MI to shock • Highest CK	Less left main as culprit lesion (4% vs 11%) Less resuscitation before admission (35% vs 49%) No significant difference in: • STEMI presentation • MI location (non-left main) • Baseline lactate • TIMI 0 flow pre-PCI	Higher STS mortality (27.9 ± 17.0 vs 20.8 ± 16.8) More cardiac arrest (67.4% vs 49.6%) Less TIMI flow 0/1 pre-PCI (49.3% vs 65.6%) No significant difference in: • STEMI • Number of diseased vessels • CK-MB troponin • Shock duration	Less anemia (51% vs 56%) Worse renal function (GFR 51.3 vs 55.7 mL/min/1.73 m^2) Similar: • Clinical presentation (slightly more rales) • Background HF medical therapy	Higher cholesterol (157 ± 47 vs 142 ± 42 mmol/L) Worse renal function (eGFR 42 vs 51 mL/min/1.73 m^2) Similar: • Clinical presentation (slightly more rales) • Background medical therapy (more calcium antagonists)

(continued on next page)

Table 1
(continued)

	Cardiogenic Shock			ADHF	
	SHOCK Registry[7,a]	**IABP-SHOCK II[8]**	**cVAD Registry[16]**	**ADHERE[6]**	**PROTECT[10]**
Hemodynamics	Lower cardiac index (1.8 ± 0.6 vs 2.2 ± 0.8) No significant difference: • PCWP, PA systolic, HR, BP, LVEF	More hypotension: (DBP 53 vs 60 mm Hg) Trend toward higher LVEF (trend 40% vs 35%)	Lower PCWP (22.8 ± 10.1 vs 31.9 ± 11.2) Higher LVEF (30.0 ± 13.2 vs 24.2 ± 11.2) No significant difference: • HR • BP • CI	Higher BP (148 vs 139 mm Hg) Higher LVEF (42.2 ± 17.3 vs 32.9 ± 15.8%)	Higher BP (SBP 127 ± 17 vs 123 ± 18 mm Hg) Higher LVEF (37 ± 14 vs 30 ± 12)
In-hospital treatment	Approach to ischemia or shock: • No difference in PTCA or thrombolysis • Fewer CABG • No difference in vasopressors, IABP, ventilation Complications: • More transfusions	Approach to ischemia or shock: • No difference in primary strategy (PCI, CABG, conservative) • Less drug eluting stents used (37% vs 50%)[b] Complications: • More moderate (but not severe) bleeding • No difference in need for renal replacement therapy • Less TIMI 3 flow post-PCI	Approach to ischemia or shock: • All underwent PCI • No significant difference in onset of MI or CS to 1st balloon inflation • Trend toward shorter duration of Impella support Complications: • More vascular complications requiring surgery (18.4% vs 9.2%) • Hematoma (10.2% vs 2.3%)	Less weight loss (−2.5 + 4.5 kg vs −3.4 + 5.0 kg) Less vasoactive therapy (24% vs 31%) • Longer time to IV vasoactive therapy (median 4.2 vs4.8 h) Fewer procedures: • CABG, IABP, PA catheter, cardioversion, cardiac catheterization (but no difference in PCI) • Less ICU or critical care use	Less weight loss (2.0 kg vs 2.6 kg) • Less diuretic (total dose day 1–7 366 mg vs 460 mg) No difference in IV vasoactive treatment

Outcome (men vs women)			
Mortality: • No significant difference in unadjusted mortality (OR 1.16, P = .252) or adjusted mortality (OR 1.03, P = .88) • No difference between men and women by strategy (no revascularization, PTCA, CABG)	Mortality: • Higher unadjusted day 1 mortality[b] • No difference at 30 d, 6 mo, 1 y	Mortality: • No difference in overall survival to discharge Other: • Better survival to discharge when Impella used before PCI in women (68.8% pre-PCI vs 24.4% post-PCI, P = .005) No difference: • ICU stay, index hospitalization duration	Mortality: • Lower unadjusted in-hospital mortality (3.8 vs 4.2%, P = .0041) • No difference after adjustment (P = .44) No difference: • Mean length of hospital stay (5.9 ± 5.3 vs 5.8 ± 6.0 d)	Mortality: • Lower age-adjusted mortality at 180-d (15.8% vs 18.5%; P = .01) • No difference after multivariable risk adjustment Other: • Longer hospitalization (11.04 ± 7.8 vs 10.65 ± 8.86 d, P = .024) No difference: • HF rehospitalization or death at 60 d • Worsening creatinine or persistent renal impairment

Abbreviations: ADHF, acute decompensated heart failure; CABG, coronary artery bypass graft; CI, cardiac index; CK-MB, creatinine kinase-muscle/brain; COPD, chronic obstructive pulmonary disease; CS, cardiogenic shock; cVAD, Catheter-Based Ventricular Assist Device (Registry); DBP, diastolic blood pressure; eGFR - estimated glomerular filtration rate; HF, heart failure; HR, heart rate; HTN, hypertension; IABP, intraaortic balloon pump; ICU, intensive care unit; LVEF, left ventricular ejection fraction; mg, milligram; MI, myocardial infarction; PA catheter, pulmonary artery catheter; PCI, percutaneous coronary intervention; PCWP, pulmonary capillary wedge pressure; PTCA, percutaneous transluminal coronary angioplasty; SBP, systolic blood pressure; STEMI, ST segment elevation myocardial infarction; STS, Society of Thoracic Surgeons; TIMI, Thrombolysis in Myocardial Infarction.

[a] SHOCK registry, data are from the cohort with predominant LV failure.
[b] No longer a predictor after stepwise regression analysis.

compared with men, women had a higher CVP (16 mm Hg vs 14 mm Hg) but, otherwise, findings were similar and consistent with severe decompensated HF. Women and men received intensive medical treatment, including vasoactive therapies, with no significant difference in their use (nitroprusside 48% vs 46%; dobutamine or milrinone 51% vs 52%, respectively). These therapies were equally well tolerated with significant improvements in hemodynamic profile and similar mean arterial blood pressure (73 mm Hg vs 74 mm Hg) at discharge. Moreover, prognosis, including all-cause mortality, and HF hospitalization were comparable between men and women. Taken together, these data suggest that women with ADHF tolerate and respond favorably to aggressive inpatient therapies. It may then be that, in the absence of hemodynamic data, there are perceived differences in hemodynamic tolerability between women and men. It is also possible that women report a historical lack of tolerability to therapies, thereby affecting treatment decisions.

Procedure-Oriented Care

Concerns have been raised about discrepancies in access to procedure-oriented care among hospitalized patients with advanced HF. When considering this issue, one must address both accessibility and outcomes. For example, women admitted with HF are consistently less likely to undergo coronary angiography.[6,21] Interestingly, among those patients who underwent catheterization in ADHERE, the rates of percutaneous coronary intervention (PCI) were not significantly different.

In the SHOCK registry, women and men were equally likely to undergo coronary angiography and PCI, and women derived equal benefit to their male counterparts.[7] However, although angiography was not mandated in the SHOCK registry, these patients were presenting at sites where angiography was readily available. In a real-world analysis of 9750 participants (44.1% women) presenting with acute myocardial infarction complicated by cardiogenic shock, women were significantly less likely to present at a site capable of revascularization, leading to lower rates of revascularization in unadjusted analysis (odds ratio [OR] 0.68, P <.001), suggesting that discrepancies still exist.[22]

In terms of surgical interventions, despite similar coronary anatomy with a predominance of 3-vessel disease in the SHOCK registry, women were less likely to undergo coronary artery bypass grafting (CABG). One reason may be the perception that women derive less benefit and may be at higher risk of adverse outcomes. However, in a recent analysis of the Surgical Treatment for Ischemic Heart Failure (STICH) trial, which randomized participants with coronary artery disease and LVEF less than or equal to 35% to medical therapy plus CABG versus medical therapy alone, there was no significant interaction between sex and treatment group with respect to all-cause mortality, cardiovascular mortality, cardiovascular hospitalization, and importantly surgical deaths.[23] These findings argue for gender equality in the consideration of surgical revascularization for advanced HF.

Temporary Mechanical Support for Acute Heart Failure and Cardiogenic Shock in Women

Overall trends in percutaneous MCS utilization have increased exponentially over the past decade; however, this may not be the case for women. In the United States, the use of percutaneous devices increased by 1511% between 2007 and 2011, with a decline in mortality.[24] Unfortunately, not only were women underrepresented but there was a trend toward decreased use among women over time.[24]

These findings raise several questions. First, is percutaneous support equally feasible? Second, do women derive the same benefit? Third, are they at increased risk of complications?

To answer the first question, in the INTERMACS registry there were no significant gender-based differences in the use of intraaortic balloon pumps (IABPs), extracorporeal membrane oxygenation (ECMO), and percutaneous left ventricular assist devices (LVADs), suggesting that it is equally feasible, although cannula size may affect decision-making.[9]

One must then consider whether women achieve the same benefit from this support. In a propensity score analysis of patients undergoing high-risk PCI with LVEF less than 35%, more than half of whom presented with NYHA class IV symptoms, women derived equal benefit from Impella (ABIOMED, Massachusetts, USA) support with similar in-hospital and 30-day survival.[17] Moreover, among patients presenting with cardiogenic shock in the Catheter-Based Ventricular Assist Device (cVAD) Registry, women who received an Impella 2.5 before PCI had significantly better survival to discharge compared with when it was implemented post-PCI (68.8% vs 24.2%, P = .005), a finding that did not reach statistical significance among the men in the study.[16] Taken together, these data suggest equal, if not better, outcomes among women who receive percutaneous mechanical support.

In this context, the final question is whether prohibitive complications limit the use of percutaneous support for women. Although in the cVAD Registry there was a slight increase in vascular complications in women and a nonsignificant trend toward more bleeding, no significant differences in stroke, renal failure, or device malfunction were observed. Furthermore, in the propensity scored analysis previously described, men experienced more in-hospital complications (41.7% vs 20.8%, P <.01).

Venoarterial Extracorporeal Membrane Oxygenation: Opportunities for Women Presenting in Cardiogenic Shock

Given the increased acuity (INTERMACS 1 and 2) and higher proportion of nonischemic causes among women, Veno-arterial-ECMO may present a unique opportunity for salvage therapy or bridge to decision in women, especially when myocardial recovery is possible.[25] This opportunity might be particularly advantageous to women for several reasons. First, women presenting with ischemic cardiogenic shock are more likely to have a de novo presentation (first myocardial infarction) with the opportunity for recovery after revascularization. Second, VA-ECMO has been used for peripartum cardiomyopathy either as bridge to recovery, LVAD, or transplant. Among 10 women who were supported on peripheral VA-ECMO for a severe peripartum cardiomyopathy, 3 were successfully weaned after myocardial recovery.[26] Unfortunately, complications remain prohibitively high and are associated with poor outcomes. In the same study, all 5 participants with complications (limb ischemia, refractory pulmonary edema, bleeding, and infection) died.

Concluding Thoughts on Advanced Inpatient Management of Women in the Setting of Acute Decompensated Heart Failure and Cardiogenic Shock

Compared with their male counterparts, women presenting with ADHF and cardiogenic shock are older and have more comorbidities, resulting in a higher baseline risk. Furthermore, women may be more likely to present in a critical state.[4,27,28] Despite this, prognoses for appropriately treated women remains favourable. Women may derive even greater benefit from short-term mechanical support, allowing for stabilization in the setting of higher acuity at presentation. Moreover, temporary mechanical support represents a unique window of opportunity for myocardial recovery. Unfortunately, women remain underrepresented in trials and registries and are likely undertreated, highlighting the urgent need to increase awareness and utilization of these therapies for appropriately selected candidates.

PART 2: CHRONIC MANAGEMENT OF ADVANCED HEART FAILURE

Advanced HF, defined as American College of Cardiology and American Heart Association stage D, represents the end-stage of a chronic and debilitating disease process. In the United States alone, this condition affects 200,000 people with an annual transition rate from stage C to D of 4.5% per year, with a similar rate of progression among men and women.[29] Individuals with stage D HF have marked dyspnea, fatigue, or other signs and symptoms of hypoperfusion on maximally tolerated medical therapy. In general, referral to advanced HF specialists is underutilized[30] but this is amplified in women who are more likely to be cared for by a primary care physician rather than a cardiologist.[31]

Although novel pharmacotherapies have improved the prognosis in advanced HF, the ultimate trajectory remains downward, with a 5-year survival of 20%.[3] There are conflicting data on gender differences and mortality in the advanced HF population. Although earlier literature suggested better survival among women,[32] more contemporary findings, indicate women have a higher adjusted risk of death.[33] Importantly, data from the United Network for Organ Sharing indicate that, compared with their male counterparts, women listed in status 1 have higher mortality, whereas those in status 2 are at lower risk of death.[28]

Given the overall trajectory and ultimate prognosis among patients with HF, and the potential life-prolonging advanced therapy options in a subset of these individuals, it is important for patients to be referred to HF specialists before they progress to end-stage disease, at which point end-organ damage (eg, renal failure) may preclude these options. The 3 main advanced therapy strategies are LVAD, heart transplant, and continuous infusion of intravenous inotrope therapy for symptom palliation. See later discussion of LVADs and inotropes. (See discussion of the complexities of heart transplantation in women in Ayesha Hasan and Michelle M. Kittleson's article, "Heart Transplantation in Women," in this issue.)

Long-Term Left Ventricular Assist Device Therapies in Women

Durable MCS with LVADs is an alternative to heart transplantation that has dramatically changed treatment of advanced HF. LVADs are surgically implanted heart pumps that are powered by external batteries and enable patients with advanced HF to return home. The current generation of LVADs are continuous-flow devices that can be used either as destination therapy in the nontransplant candidate or as a bridge to transplantation.

Initial LVADs were large, pulsatile pumps and, owing to body-size constraints, the early trials had 0% to 20% female representation.[34–36] In a single-center cohort study of early (1990–2002) bridge-to-transplant LVADs, women had a statistically significant decrease in posttransplant survival compared with men at 5 years (50.9% and 85.2% in women and men, respectively). Multivariate analysis of this population showed that the gender difference was driven by a greater severity of illness at time of LVAD implant in women.[37] In a review of the earliest LVAD studies with the large pulsatile HeartMate (HM) (Abbott Laboratories, Illinois, USA) XVE, women were more likely to develop severe right HF requiring a right ventricular assist device support, with an OR of 4.5.[38] Therefore, in these early days of durable LVADs, the gender bias, which was partially due to body size, may have been justifiably driven by significant differences in outcomes.

Advances in technology have led to smaller continuous-flow pumps, eliminating some of the anatomic limitations to LVAD support in women. As a result, their representation in clinical trials and in INTERMACS has increased, although they remain the minority, representing only 22% to 30%.[39,40]

There are 3 contemporary, continuous-flow LVADs in use. The HMII is an axial flow device with a centrifugal pump and is the most commonly used durable LVAD in the United States. The HeartWare LVAD (HVAD) (Medtronic, Minneapolis, USA) is an intrapericardial centrifugal-flow LVAD. It is a smaller pump than the HMII and can be implanted in patients with a body surface area as low as 1.2 m². Finally, the newest continuous-flow LVAD is the HM3. This is a fully magnetically levitated centrifugal continuous-flow pump that has wide blood-flow passages that are frictionless, thus redcing shear stress. This pump is programmed to have an intrinsic fixed artificial pulse to reduce stasis. The HMII and HVAD are approved for destination therapy and bridge-to-transplant indications, whereas the HM3 is approved for bridge-to-transplant only. Major risks of these devices are stroke (both ischemic and hemorrhagic), bleeding (specifically gastrointestinal bleeding), and device-related infections.

Despite the evolution of these pumps, there continues to be a gender difference in outcomes. An initial review of the HMII and HVAD bridge-to-transplant studies found that there was no difference in survival of men versus women during the first 6 to 18 months of LVAD support.[39,41] However, a closer look at the INTERMACS registry from 1994 to 2012, reveals that women had a higher rate of major adverse events than men (OR 2.01, 95% CI 1.56–2.53, P <.001). This was driven by stroke and in-hospital mortality (52.3% vs 40.8%).[42]

One of the most devastating complications from LVAD support is stroke. In the initial HVAD trial, the first 48-hour postimplant stroke rate, both ischemic and hemorrhagic, trended higher in women (9.4%) versus men (3.0%) but did not reach statistical significance.[39] In the HMII bridge-to-transplant study, women suffered more hemorrhagic stroke than men.[41] In a cohort of more than 1800 LVAD participants, compared with men, women were at increased risk of stroke (HR 1.6 for all stroke and 2.2 for hemorrhagic stroke),[43] although contemporary generalizability is limited by inclusion of the early pulsatile LVADs. Recent INTERMACS data looking at only continuous-flow LVADs demonstrated an overall stroke risk of 10.57%.[44] Importantly, female gender was a preimplant risk factor for this complication (HR 1.51). Other preimplant predictors included systolic blood pressure, IABP, and heparin-induced thrombocytopenia (HIT), with only HIT having a more robust HR of 3.68.[44] In another study, among 110 participants implanted with either an HMII or HVAD, the risk of stroke was also higher for women than men (HR of 3.1, 95% CI 1.4–6.9, P = .007); however, survival rates were similar.[45] Importantly, the newest LVAD, HM3, has a much reduced overall risk of stroke and may thus be particularly advantageous to women.[40]

Other major complications include bleeding and infection. In a single-center review of 375 participants with continuous-flow LVAD, women experienced a 60% higher hazard of bleeding than their male counterparts. Importantly, however, the results were driven by mucosal bleeding, which is generally not life-threatening.[46] In terms of infection, women have fared better with either similar or lower rates of this complication,[39,41] which may be related to body size.

Finally, LVAD use in women continues to be plagued by earlier right HF for which, currently, there are few durable support options. Moreover, outcomes among patients requiring biventricular support remain poor, including when used as a bridge to transplant.[47] The increased right HF is likely due women presenting with more advanced disease, thus highlighting the need for earlier referral to HF specialists.

Palliative Inotropes

Patients with advanced HF have symptoms that are due to chronic hypoperfusion and congestion. Continuous infusion of inotropes improves both hemodynamics and symptoms. These medications are used (1) to stabilize patients waiting for heart transplant, (2) to optimize patients before LVAD implantation, or (3) as palliation. Historically, outcomes in patients on inotropes have been poor, with survival ranges from 40% to 74% at 6 months[48–51] and 25% at 1 year.[36] In these earlier trials, high doses were used in the absence of standard neurohormonal blockade or defibrillators. More recent retrospective data suggest a better 1-year survival of 47.6%. Importantly, these participants were on lower doses of inotropes, many were on standard HF therapies, and 90% had a defibrillator, Similar to other advanced HF trials, only 25.8% were women.[52] To date, there have been no studies to specifically look at gender differences on outcomes or use of palliative inotropes.

Psychosocial Issues Impacting the Treatment of Advanced Heart Failure in Women

Although studies both in the acute and chronic HF setting suggest similar benefit to advanced therapies among women and men, there are significant epidemiologic and societal considerations that play a role in women's acceptance of and candidacy for advanced therapies. In a study of gender differences after implantable cardioverter defibrillator implantation, women were more likely to live alone and less likely to be married or living in a common law relationship.[53] This presents a barrier because most MCS programs require the patient to have a dedicated caregiver. It is of interest to note that when patient refusal was removed from the equation, the gender bias in transplant listing disappeared.[54] This leads to the final point, which merits great attention but is notoriously difficult to study, namely the gender differences in the perception and acceptance of advanced therapies by both patients and their physicians. Clearly, as work progresses toward improving the mechanics of device therapies, an urgent call-to-arms is needed that addresses the psychosocial barriers that will ultimately limit the use of these life-preserving therapies in women.

Summary: Toward Improving Outcomes in Women with Advanced Heart Failure

Women with advanced HF are afflicted by a similar disease process and resultant poor outcomes as are their male counterparts. Although women remain underrepresented in clinical trials of both short-term and durable MCS, the sum total of evidence suggests that they derive equal benefit to men. In the acute setting, it is now clear that early revascularization for ischemia and aggressive use of percutaneous support is feasible and results in favorable outcomes. Unfortunately, in the setting of chronic HF, women tend to present later in the disease process, often with more comorbidities, higher INTERMACS status, and more biventricular failure. Furthermore, they are more likely to present with a preserved ejection fraction. These factors affect the ability to provide device therapies, which are often less efficacious in these settings. Importantly, there is an urgent need to improve timely referral to overcome the limitations of irreversible end-organ dysfunction. Finally, the psychosocial situation unique to women must be addressed with the goal of increasing patient acceptance and candidacy.

REFERENCES

1. Fang JC, Ewald GA, Allen LA, et al. Advanced (stage D) heart failure: a statement from the Heart Failure Society of America Guidelines Committee. J Card Fail 2015;21(6):519–34.
2. Ponikowski P, Voors AA, Anker SD, et al. 2016 ESC Guidelines for the diagnosis and treatment of acute and chronic heart failure: the Task Force for the diagnosis and treatment of acute and chronic heart failure of the European Society of Cardiology (ESC) Developed with the special contribution of the Heart Failure Association (HFA) of the ESC. Eur Heart J 2016;37(27):2129–200.
3. Yancy CW, Jessup M, Bozkurt B, et al. 2013 ACCF/AHA guideline for the management of heart failure: executive summary: a report of the American College of Cardiology Foundation/American Heart Association Task Force on practice guidelines. Circulation 2013;128(16):1810–52.
4. Shin JJ, Hamad E, Murthy S, et al. Heart failure in women. Clin Cardiol 2012;35(3):172–7.
5. Fonarow GC, Abraham WT, Albert NM, et al. Age- and gender-related differences in quality of care and outcomes of patients hospitalized with heart failure (from OPTIMIZE-HF). Am J Cardiol 2009;104(1):107–15.
6. Galvao M, Kalman J, DeMarco T, et al. Gender differences in in-hospital management and outcomes in patients with decompensated heart failure: analysis from the Acute Decompensated Heart Failure National Registry (ADHERE). J Card Fail 2006;12(2):100–7.
7. Wong SC, Sleeper LA, Monrad ES, et al. Absence of gender differences in clinical outcomes in patients with cardiogenic shock complicating acute myocardial infarction. A report from the SHOCK Trial Registry. J Am Coll Cardiol 2001;38(5):1395–401.
8. Fengler K, Fuernau G, Desch S, et al. Gender differences in patients with cardiogenic shock complicating myocardial infarction: a substudy of the

IABP-SHOCK II-trial. Clin Res Cardiol 2015;104(1):71–8.

9. Cowger J, Shah P, Stulak J, et al. INTERMACS profiles and modifiers: heterogeneity of patient classification and the impact of modifiers on predicting patient outcome. J Heart Lung Transplant 2016;35(4):440–8.

10. Meyer S, van der Meer P, Massie BM, et al. Sex-specific acute heart failure phenotypes and outcomes from PROTECT. Eur J Heart Fail 2013;15(12):1374–81.

11. Mullens W, Abrahams Z, Sokos G, et al. Gender differences in patients admitted with advanced decompensated heart failure. Am J Cardiol 2008;102(4):454–8.

12. Woodfield SL, Lundergan CF, Reiner JS, et al. Gender and acute myocardial infarction: is there a different response to thrombolysis? J Am Coll Cardiol 1997;29(1):35–42.

13. Vaccarino V, Parsons L, Every NR, et al. Sex-based differences in early mortality after myocardial infarction. National Registry of Myocardial Infarction 2 Participants. N Engl J Med 1999;341(4):217–25.

14. Malacrida R, Genoni M, Maggioni AP, et al. A comparison of the early outcome of acute myocardial infarction in women and men. The Third International Study of Infarct Survival Collaborative Group. N Engl J Med 1998;338(1):8–14.

15. Karlson BW, Herlitz J, Hartford M. Prognosis in myocardial infarction in relation to gender. Am Heart J 1994;128(3):477–83.

16. Joseph SM, Brisco MA, Colvin M, et al. Women with cardiogenic shock derive greater benefit from early mechanical circulatory support: an update from the cVAD registry. J Interv Cardiol 2016;29(3):248–56.

17. Doshi R, Singh A, Jauhar R, et al. Gender difference with the use of percutaneous left ventricular assist device in patients undergoing complex high-risk percutaneous coronary intervention: from pVAD Working Group. Eur Heart J Acute Cardiovasc Care 2018. 2048872617745790. [Epub ahead of print].

18. Cuffe MS, Califf RM, Adams KF Jr, et al. Short-term intravenous milrinone for acute exacerbation of chronic heart failure: a randomized controlled trial. JAMA 2002;287(12):1541–7.

19. Konstam MA, Gheorghiade M, Burnett JC Jr, et al. Effects of oral tolvaptan in patients hospitalized for worsening heart failure: the EVEREST outcome trial. JAMA 2007;297(12):1319–31.

20. Felker GM, Lee KL, Bull DA, et al. Diuretic strategies in patients with acute decompensated heart failure. N Engl J Med 2011;364(9):797–805.

21. Nieminen MS, Harjola VP, Hochadel M, et al. Gender related differences in patients presenting with acute heart failure. Results from EuroHeart Failure Survey II. Eur J Heart Fail 2008;10(2):140–8.

22. Abdel-Qadir HM, Ivanov J, Austin PC, et al. Sex differences in the management and outcomes of Ontario patients with cardiogenic shock complicating acute myocardial infarction. Can J Cardiol 2013;29(6):691–6.

23. Pina IL, Zheng Q, She L, et al. Sex difference in patients with ischemic heart failure undergoing surgical revascularization: results from the STICH Trial (Surgical Treatment for Ischemic Heart Failure). Circulation 2018;137(8):771–80.

24. Stretch R, Sauer CM, Yuh DD, et al. National trends in the utilization of short-term mechanical circulatory support: incidence, outcomes, and cost analysis. J Am Coll Cardiol 2014;64(14):1407–15.

25. Tarzia V, Bortolussi G, Bianco R, et al. Extracorporeal life support in cardiogenic shock: impact of acute versus chronic etiology on outcome. J Thorac Cardiovasc Surg 2015;150(2):333–40.

26. Bouabdallaoui N, Demondion P, Leprince P, et al. Short-term mechanical circulatory support for cardiogenic shock in severe peripartum cardiomyopathy: La Pitie-Salpetriere experience. Interact Cardiovasc Thorac Surg 2017;25(1):52–6.

27. Magnussen C, Bernhardt AM, Ojeda FM, et al. Gender differences and outcomes in left ventricular assist device support: The European Registry for Patients with Mechanical Circulatory Support. J Heart Lung Transplant 2018;37(1):61–70.

28. Hsich EM, Naftel DC, Myers SL, et al. Should women receive left ventricular assist device support?: findings from INTERMACS. Circ Heart Fail 2012;5(2):234–40.

29. Kalogeropoulos AP, Samman-Tahhan A, Hedley JS, et al. Progression to stage D heart failure among outpatients with stage C Heart failure and reduced ejection fraction. JACC Heart Fail 2017;5(7):528–37.

30. Peura JL, Colvin-Adams M, Francis GS, et al. Recommendations for the use of mechanical circulatory support: device strategies and patient selection: a scientific statement from the American Heart Association. Circulation 2012;126(22):2648–67.

31. Petrie MC, Dawson NF, Murdoch DR, et al. Failure of women's hearts. Circulation 1999;99(17):2334–41.

32. Adams KF Jr, Sueta CA, Gheorghiade M, et al. Gender differences in survival in advanced heart failure. Insights from the FIRST study. Circulation 1999;99(14):1816–21.

33. Weidner G, Zahn D, Mendell NR, et al. Patients' sex and emotional support as predictors of death and clinical deterioration in the waiting for a new heart study: results from the 1-year follow-up. Prog Transplant 2011;21(2):106–14.

34. Copeland JG, Smith RG, Arabia FA, et al. Cardiac replacement with a total artificial heart as a bridge to transplantation. N Engl J Med 2004;351(9):859–67.

35. Frazier OH, Rose EA, Oz MC, et al. Multicenter clinical evaluation of the HeartMate vented electric left ventricular assist system in patients awaiting heart transplantation. J Thorac Cardiovasc Surg 2001; 122(6):1186–95.

36. Rose EA, Gelijns AC, Moskowitz AJ, et al. Long-term use of a left ventricular assist device for end-stage heart failure. N Engl J Med 2001;345(20):1435–43.

37. Morgan JA, Weinberg AD, Hollingsworth KW, et al. Effect of gender on bridging to transplantation and posttransplantation survival in patients with left ventricular assist devices. J Thorac Cardiovasc Surg 2004;127(4):1193–5.

38. Ochiai Y, McCarthy PM, Smedira NG, et al. Predictors of severe right ventricular failure after implantable left ventricular assist device insertion: analysis of 245 patients. Circulation 2002;106(12 Suppl 1): I198–202.

39. Birks EJ, McGee EC Jr, Aaronson KD, et al. An examination of survival by sex and race in the HeartWare Ventricular Assist Device for the Treatment of Advanced Heart Failure (ADVANCE) Bridge to Transplant (BTT) and continued access protocol trials. J Heart Lung Transplant 2015;34(6):815–24.

40. Mehra MR, Naka Y, Uriel N, et al. A fully magnetically levitated circulatory pump for advanced heart failure. N Engl J Med 2017;376(5):440–50.

41. Bogaev RC, Pamboukian SV, Moore SA, et al. Comparison of outcomes in women versus men using a continuous-flow left ventricular assist device as a bridge to transplantation. J Heart Lung Transplant 2011;30(5):515–22.

42. McIlvennan CK, Lindenfeld J, Kao DP. Sex differences and in-hospital outcomes in patients undergoing mechanical circulatory support implantation. J Heart Lung Transplant 2017;36(1):82–90.

43. Parikh NS, Cool J, Karas MG, et al. Stroke risk and mortality in patients with ventricular assist devices. Stroke 2016;47(11):2702–6.

44. Acharya D, Loyaga-Rendon R, Morgan CJ, et al. INTERMACS analysis of stroke during support with continuous-flow left ventricular assist devices: risk factors and outcomes. JACC Heart Fail 2017;5(10): 703–11.

45. Morris AA, Pekarek A, Wittersheim K, et al. Gender differences in the risk of stroke during support with continuous-flow left ventricular assist device. J Heart Lung Transplant 2015;34(12):1570–7.

46. Yavar Z, Cowger JA, Moainie SL, et al. Bleeding complication rates are higher in females after continuous-flow left ventricular assist device implantation. ASAIO J 2017. [Epub ahead of print].

47. Grimm JC, Sciortino CM, Magruder JT, et al. Outcomes in patients bridged with univentricular and biventricular devices in the modern era of heart transplantation. Ann Thorac Surg 2016;102(1): 102–8.

48. Hauptman PJ, Mikolajczak P, George A, et al. Chronic inotropic therapy in end-stage heart failure. Am Heart J 2006;152(6):1096.e1-8.

49. Stevenson LW. Clinical use of inotropic therapy for heart failure: looking backward or forward? Part II: chronic inotropic therapy. Circulation 2003;108(4): 492–7.

50. Hershberger RE, Nauman D, Walker TL, et al. Care processes and clinical outcomes of continuous outpatient support with inotropes (COSI) in patients with refractory endstage heart failure. J Card Fail 2003;9(3):180–7.

51. Gorodeski EZ, Chu EC, Reese JR, et al. Prognosis on chronic dobutamine or milrinone infusions for stage D heart failure. Circ Heart Fail 2009;2(4): 320–4.

52. Hashim T, Sanam K, Revilla-Martinez M, et al. Clinical characteristics and outcomes of intravenous inotropic therapy in advanced heart failure. Circ Heart Fail 2015;8(5):880–6.

53. Lauck SB, Sawatzky R, Johnson JL, et al. Sex is associated with differences in individual trajectories of change in social health after implantable cardioverter-defibrillator. Circ Cardiovasc Qual Outcomes 2015;8(2 Suppl 1):S21–30.

54. Aaronson KD, Schwartz JS, Goin JE, et al. Sex differences in patient acceptance of cardiac transplant candidacy. Circulation 1995;91(11):2753–61.

Implantable Cardioverter-Defibrillators and Cardiac Resynchronization Therapy in Women

Maya T. Ignaszewski, MD[a],*,
Stacie L. Daugherty, MD, MSPH[b],
Andrea M. Russo, MD, FHRS[a]

KEYWORDS

- Implantable cardioverter-defibrillator (ICD) • Cardiac resynchronization therapy (CRT)
- Gender differences • Heart failure

KEY POINTS

- Gaps exist in the utilization of implantable cardioverter-defibrillators (ICDs) and cardiac resynchronization therapy (CRT) mainly among women
- Landmark ICD trials were underpowered to demonstrate benefit of therapy in women due to low enrollment.
- Despite clear benefit among women receiving CRT, eligible women are less likely to receive this therapy.
- Guideline recommendations remain gender neutral for implantation of ICD and CRT despite studies suggesting women benefit more than men.

IMPLANTABLE CARDIOVERTER-DEFIBRILLATOR THERAPY

Epidemiology of Sudden Cardiac Arrest and Sudden Cardiac Death in Women and Men

It is estimated that 400,000 to 460,000 cases of sudden cardiac death (SCD) occur annually in the United States,[1] with the incidence of SCD approximately 3 times higher in men than in women.[2] There are gender differences in the epidemiology of SCD although the absolute incidence increases with age in both men and women.[3] Women have a lower incidence of SCD than men at any age even after adjusting for coronary heart disease risk factors, with a 10-year to 20-year lag seen in women.[4] Two-thirds of women who presented with unexpected SCD occurred in the setting of no known coronary heart disease in comparison with 50% in men.[3] Among sudden cardiac arrest (SCA) survivors, women were significantly less likely to carry a diagnosis of structural heart disease compared with men.[5]

Gender differences also exist in the initial presenting rhythm in patients presenting with out-of-hospital cardiac arrest. Studies have shown that men are more likely to have shockable rhythms, including ventricular tachycardia (VT) or ventricular fibrillation (VF), whereas women are more likely to present with pulseless electrical activity or asystole.[6,7] Women more frequently presented with SCA at home, however, and were more likely to survive to hospital discharge than men.[7]

Implantable Cardioverter-Defibrillator Trials: The Evidence by Gender

Randomized clinical trials have demonstrated the efficacy of ICDs in the primary and secondary

[a] Cooper University Hospital, 1 Cooper Plaza, 3 Dorrance, Camden, NJ 08103, USA; [b] University of Colorado, Academic Office 1, 12631 East 17th Avenue B130, Aurora, CO 80045, USA
* Corresponding author.
E-mail address: mayaigna@gmail.com

Heart Failure Clin 15 (2019) 109–125
https://doi.org/10.1016/j.hfc.2018.08.011
1551-7136/19/© 2018 Elsevier Inc. All rights reserved.

Table 1
Summary of primary prevention implantable cardioverter-defibrillator trials

Study (Year)	Patients Enrolled = n (%)	Inclusion Criteria	Treatment Arms	Outcomes
MADIT-I (1996)	Men: 184 (92%) Women: 16 (8%)	Post–acute MI, NSVT, LVEF ≤35%, NYHA classes I–III	ICD vs conventional therapy	• 54% ↓ in risk of death in ICD group
MUSTT (1999)	Men: 1265 (84%) Women: 233 (16%)	LVEF ≤40% and CAD, NYHA I–III, NSVT, or SVT induced in EPS	OMT ± ICD vs no EP- guided therapy	• 28% ↓ rate of SCA/ SCD • 21% ↓ in overall mortality at 5 y (P = .06) in EP-guided therapy and ICD vs no EP-guided therapy
MADIT-II (2002)	Men: 1047 (85%) Women: 192 (16%)	LVEF ≤30%, >l mo post-MI	ICD vs conventional therapy	• 12% ↓ in overall death at 1 y, 28% at 2 y, and 28% at 3 y (P = .007) • Overall 31% ↓ risk reduction of death in ICD group
DEFINITE (2004)	Men: 326 (71%) Women: 132 (29%)	NICM, LVEF ≤35%, NSVT or >10 PVC on 24-h Holter, symptomatic HF	NICM standard medical therapy ± ICD	• ICD ↓ risk of arrhythmic death (HR 0.20; P = .006) • Reduction in risk of death from any cause (HR 0.65; P = .08)
SCD-HeFT (2005)	Men: 1941 (77%) Women: 588 (23%)	NYHA classes II–III, LVEF ≤35%	ICD vs amiodarone vs placebo	• 23% ↓ risk of death with ICD and ARR in mortality of 7.2% vs placebo

Abbreviations: AMI, acute myocardial infarction; ARR, absolute risk reduction; EP, electrophysiology; EPS, electrophysiology study; HR, heart rate; MI, myocardial infarction; NICM, non-ischemic cardiomyopathy; NSVT, non-sustained ventricular tachycardia; PVC, premature ventricular contraction; RBBB, right bundle branch block; SVT, supra ventricular tachycardia.

prevention of SCD. **Tables 1** and **2** summarize the major primary and secondary prevention trials with representation of women enrolled in each trial. The American College of Cardiology (ACC)/American Heart Association (AHA)/Heart Rhythm Society (HRS) guidelines include indications for ICD implantation for primary prevention and secondary prevention of SCD for both ischemic and nonischemic cardiomyopathy (**Figs. 1** and **2**)[8] and are based on the multicenter clinical trials described in **Tables 1** and **2**. Current ICD guidelines make no distinction between recommendations for ICD therapy by gender. Due to the small number of women enrolled, caution is needed with interpretation of post hoc analyses because these trials were underpowered to demonstrate a benefit of ICD therapy in women. This highlights the importance of including enough women in clinical trials to assure that results can be extrapolated to both genders.

Gender Differences in Comorbidities Among Implantable Cardioverter-Defibrillator Populations

A large population-based study revealed that women who underwent primary prevention ICD implantation were more likely to have heart failure (HF), nonischemic cardiomyopathy, and worse New York Heart Association (NYHA) functional class and to receive cardiac resynchronization therapy-defibrillator (CRT-D).[9] The influence of gender on arrhythmia characteristics and outcomes of the MUSTT trial were analyzed and found that women were older and more likely to have history of HF, a myocardial infarction (MI) within 6 months, and recent angina prior to enrollment than men.[10] The MADIT-II trial demonstrated that women were more likely to have hypertension, advanced HF, left bundle branch block (LBBB), and diabetes.[11]

Table 2
Summary of secondary prevention implantable cardioverter-defibrillator trials

Study (Year)	Patients Enrolled = n (%)	Inclusion Criteria	Treatment Arms	Outcomes
AVID (1999)	Men: 813 (80%) Women: 203 (20%)	Resuscitation from VF, VT with syncope, sustained VT with LVEF ≤40% and hemodynamic compromise, excluded if within 72 h of MI, cardiac surgery, or electrolyte imbalance	ICD vs amiodarone or sotalol	• ↓ death rates of 39%, 27% and 31% at 1 y, 2 y, and 3 y, respectively in ICD group vs medication therapy alone (P<.02)
CASH (2000)	Men: 230 (80%) Women: 58 (20%)	Resuscitated arrest from VT/VF, excluded if within 72 h of MI, cardiac surgery or electrolyte imbalance	ICD vs amiodarone or metoprolol	• 23% ↓ all-cause mortality in ICD vs medical treatment with amiodarone or metoprolol (P = .081)
CIDS (2000)	Men: 560 (85%) Women: 99 (15%)	Documented VF, out of hospital arrest requiring defibrillation, sustained VT causing syncope, VT >150 BPM with presyncope, LVEF ≤35%, syncope with induced monomorphic VT	ICD vs amiodarone	• 20% RRR in all-cause mortality in ICD group (P = .081) • 33% ↓ in arrhythmic mortality in group with ICD compared with amiodarone (P = .005)

The baseline characteristics of 5 studies were pooled, including MUSTT, MADIT-II, DEFINITE, SCD-HeFT, and COMPANION trials, and found that nonwhite race, higher NYHA class and greater use of diuretics was more prevalent among women (**Table 3**).[12] In general, women with ICD indications were older and were more likely to have advanced noncardiac conditions, rendering them "higher risk" at the time of enrollment. It is postulated that these more advanced conditions predispose women to increased noncardiac and nonarrhythmic mortality, which may influence the benefit of ICD therapy in women.[13]

Gender Differences in Implantable Cardioverter-Defibrillator Mortality Benefit

Perhaps the most widely analyzed gender difference in the ICD literature is the effect of devices on mortality. The data are conflicting; several trials, such as DEFINITE and SCD-HeFT, reported mortality benefit for men but not for women for primary prevention of SCD.[14,15] After adjustment for differences in baseline characteristics, overall mortality in SCD-HeFT was lower in women than in men (**Fig. 3**).[16] MUSTT and MADIT-II showed no statistically significant difference in mortality among men and women in the standard medical therapy arm versus the treatment arm.[11,17] In contrast, a study linked data from hospitals included in the Get With The Guidelines–Heart Failure (GWTG-HF) registry with data from Centers for Medicare and Medicaid Services and found improved survival rates among female and male patients with reduced left ventricular ejection fraction (LVEF) with primary prevention ICDs.[18]

Several large meta-analyses of randomized controlled trials for primary prevention of SCD were conducted as a result of this inconsistent evidence. Five clinical trials (MADIT-II, COMPANION, DEFINITE, DINAMIT, and SCD-HeFT) that included 6405 patients, of whom 1575 (25%) were women, were examined and found that risk of death from any cause was reduced by 26% in

A

COR	LOE	Recommendations for Primary Prevention of SCD in Patients With Ischemic Heart Disease
I	A	In patients with LVEF of 35% or less that is due to ischemic heart disease who are at least 40 d' post-MI and at least 90 d post-revascularization, and with NYHA class II or III HF despite GDMT, an ICD is recommended if meaningful survival of greater than 1 y is expected.
I	A	In patients with LVEF of 30% or less that is due to ischemic heart disease who are at least 40 d' post-MI and at least 90 d post-revascularization, and with NYHA class I HF despite GDMT, an ICD is recommended if meaningful survival of greater than 1 y is expected.
I	B-R	In patients with NSVT due to prior MI, LVEF of 40% or less and inducible sustained VT or VF at electrophysiological study, an ICD is recommended if meaningful survival of greater than 1 y is expected.
IIa	B-NR	In nonhospitalized patients with NYHA class IV symptoms who are candidates for cardiac transplantation or an LVAD, an ICD is reasonable if meaningful survival of greater than 1 y is expected.
III: No Benefit	C-EO	An ICD is not indicated for NYHA class IV patients with medication-refractory HF who are not also candidates for cardiac transplantation, an LVAD, or a CRT defibrillator that incorporates both pacing and defibrillation capabilities.

B

COR	LOE	Recommendations for Primary Prevention of SCD in Patients With NICM
I	A	In patients with NICM, HF with NYHA class II–III symptoms and an LVEF of 35% or less, despite GDMT, an ICD is recommended if meaningful survival of greater than 1 y is expected.
IIa	B-NR	In patients with NICM due to a *Lamin A/C* mutation who have 2 or more risk factors (NSVT, LVEF <45%, nonmissense mutation, and male sex), an ICD can be beneficial if meaningful survival of greater than 1 y is expected.
IIb	B-R	In patients with NICM, HF with NYHA class I symptoms and an LVEF of 35% or less, despite GDMT, an ICD may be considered if meaningful survival of greater than 1 y is expected.
III: No Benefit	C-EO	In patients with medication-refractory NYHA class IV HF who are not also candidates for cardiac transplantation, an LVAD, or a CRT defibrillator that incorporates both pacing and defibrillation capabilities, an ICD should not be implanted.

Fig. 1. 2017 AHA/ACC/HRS guidelines for primary prevention of SCD. (*A*) Primary prevention indications for patients with ischemic heart disease are summarized. (*B*) Primary prevention indications for patients with nonischemic cardiomyopathy are summarized. Class of recommendation (COR), expert opinion (EO), goal directed medical therapy (GDMT), left ventricular assist device (LVAD), non-ischemic cardiomyopathy (NICM); nonrandomized (NR); randomized (R). (*Adapted from* Al-Khatib SM, Stevenson WG, Ackerman MJ, et al. 2017 AHA/ACC/HRS Guideline for Management of Patients With Ventricular Arrhythmias and the Prevention of Sudden Cardiac Death A Report of the American College of Cardiology/American Heart Association Task Force on Clinical Practice Guidelines and the Heart Rhythm Society. Heart Rhythm; © Elsevier 2018; with permission.)

men who received ICD therapy but not among women.[19] Similarly, in a meta-analysis of 5 primary prevention trials that included both ischemic or nonischemic heart disease (MUSTT, MADIT-II, DEFINITE, SCD-HeFT, and COMPANION), no significant gender differences in overall mortality were noted (**Fig. 4**).[12] A statistically significant mortality benefit of ICD therapy was seen, however, in men but not in women (**Fig. 5**).[12]

Three secondary prevention trials (AVID, CASH, and CIDS) showed decreased rates of all-cause mortality with use of ICDs for secondary prevention[20–23] (see **Table 2**). Unfortunately, detailed analyses of secondary prevention ICD trials by gender are

A

COR	LOE	Recommendations for Secondary Prevention of SCD in Patients With Ischemic Heart Disease
I	B-R / B-NR	In patients with ischemic heart disease who either survive SCA due to VT/VF or experience hemodynamically unstable VT (LOE: B-R) or stable VT (LOE: B-NR) not due to reversible causes, an ICD is recommended if meaningful survival greater than 1 y is expected.
I	B-NR	In patients with ischemic heart disease and unexplained syncope who have inducible sustained monomorphic VT on electrophysiological study, an ICD is recommended if meaningful survival of greater than 1 y is expected.

B

COR	LOE	Recommendations for Secondary Prevention of SCD in Patients With NICM
I	B-R / B-NR	In patients with NICM who either survive SCA due to VT/VF or experience hemodynamically unstable VT (LOE: B-R) or stable VT (LOE: B-NR) not due to reversible causes, an ICD is recommended if meaningful survival greater than 1 y is expected.
IIa	B-NR	In patients with NICM who experience syncope presumed to be due to VA and who do not meet indications for a primary prevention ICD, an ICD or an electrophysiological study for risk stratification for SCD can be beneficial if meaningful survival greater than 1 y is expected.

Fig. 2. AHA/ACC/HRS 2017 guidelines for secondary prevention of SCD. (*A*) Secondary prevention indications for patients with ischemic heart disease are summarized. (*B*) Secondary prevention indications for patients with nonischemic cardiomyopathy are summarized. (Adapted from Al-Khatib SM, Stevenson WG, Ackerman MJ, et al. 2017 AHA/ACC/HRS Guideline for Management of Patients With Ventricular Arrhythmias and the Prevention of Sudden Cardiac Death A Report of the American College of Cardiology/American Heart Association Task Force on Clinical Practice Guidelines and the Heart Rhythm Society. Heart Rhythm; © Elsevier 2018; with permission.)

not available. Guidelines for ICD placement for secondary prevention include patients with ischemic or nonischemic heart disease and make no distinction by gender (see **Fig. 2**).[8] In an analysis of a Medicare cohort, although women were less likely to receive ICD therapy for a secondary prevention indication than men, the mortality benefit was significant for both genders.[23]

One of the strongest potential explanations for gender differences in outcomes with ICD therapy includes the smaller proportion of women enrolled in trials. Women represented anywhere from 8% to 29% of total patients studied. Consistently across landmark trials, the wide confidence limits of the hazard ratios for mortality benefit indicate that these studies were underpowered to detect a significant difference by gender, attributed to the low enrollment of women overall. No trial was a priori powered to detect a gender difference in mortality. Differences in ICD benefit by gender may be related to differences in baseline characteristics, age, comorbidities, or disease severity. It is also

possible that gender differences in arrhythmia substrate or hormonal differences contribute to a lower overall arrhythmic risk in women. Given the lack of strong evidence to support gender differences in ICD outcomes, current guidelines for ICD implantation for primary and secondary prevention do not vary by gender. Future studies with larger numbers of women are needed to evaluate the effectiveness of ICDs in women.

Under-Representation of Women in Implantable Cardioverter-Defibrillator Trials

As discussed previously, women represent only a small percentage of subjects enrolled in primary and secondary prevention ICD trials (see **Tables 1** and **2**). Potential reasons for under-representation of women in clinical trials include potential physician bias at the time of screening or higher rates of refusal of women who may be less willing to participate.[24] Alternatively, women may be referred less often to subspecialists who may consider trial

Table 3
Baseline characteristics of men and women enrolled in primary prevention implantable cardioverter-defibrillator trials

Baseline Characteristics of Men and Women in the Included Studies

	MUSTT[4]		MADIT-II[5]		DEFINITE[2]		SCD-HeFT[3]	
	Men (n = 1265)	Women (n = 233)	Men (n = 1040)	Women (n = 192)	Men (n = 326)	Women (n = 132)	Men (n = 1933)	Women (n = 588)
Age (y) (mean ± SD, median [range], or n [%] <70)	835 (66)	156 (67)	65 ± 10	64 ± 11	57.9	59.1	60 (52–69)	60 (50–67)
Nonwhite race	177 (14)	56 (24)[d]	110 (11)	49 (25)[d]	94 (29)	55 (42)[d]	406 (21)	182 (31)[d]
NYHA functional class >II	NR	NR	643 (63)	132 (70)	65 (20)	31 (24)	541 (28)	212 (36)
Ischemic etiology	1265 (100)	233 (100)	1040 (100)	192 (100)	0 (0)	0 (0)	1102 (57)	200 (34)[d]
Nonischemic etiology	0 (0)	0 (0)	0 (0)	0 (0)	326 (100)	132 (100)	831 (43)	388 (66)[d]
LVEF (%) (mean ± SD, median [range], or n [%] <30%)	645 (51)	103 (44)[c]	23.1 ± 5.4	23.6 ± 5.7	21 (7–35)	22 (10–35)	24 (20–30)	25 (20–30)
Prior revascularization[a]	949 (75)	149 (64)[d]	626 (60)	81 (42)[d]	0 (0)	0 (0)	1411 (73)	394 (67)
ECG parameters								
Atrial fibrillation	114 (9)	19 (8)	96 (9)	9 (5)[c]	NR	NR	329 (17)	53 (9)[d]
LBBB	63 (5)	26 (11)[d]	164 (17)	45 (25)[c]	NR	NR	NR	NR
Medication								
Angiotensin-converting enzyme inhibitor	911 (72)	177 (76)	822 (79)	136 (71)[c]	310 (95)	124 (94)	1662 (86)	476 (81)[c]
β-Blocker	455 (36)	70 (30)	655 (63)	113 (59)	277 (85)	112 (85)	1334 (69)	400 (68)
Diuretics[b]	721 (57)	154 (66)[c]	759 (73)	163 (85)[d]	NR	NR	1565 (81)	506 (86)[c]
Digoxin	696 (55)	147 (63)[c]	603 (58)	123 (64)	140 (43)	51 (39)	1314 (68)	435 (74)

Values are expressed as n (%).

Abbreviation: NR, not reported.

[a] Percutaneous or surgical coronary revascularization in MUSTT and SCD-HeFT, surgical coronary revascularization in MADIT-II.
[b] Loop diuretics in SCD-HeFT. In the other studies, type of diuretic used was not specified.
[c] P≤.05.
[d] P≤.001 for comparisons between men and women.

From Santangeli P, Pelargonio G, Dello Russo A, et al. Gender differences in clinical outcome and primary prevention defibrillator benefit in patients with severe left ventricular dysfunction: a systematic review and meta-analysis. Heart Rhythm 2010;7(7):879; with permission.

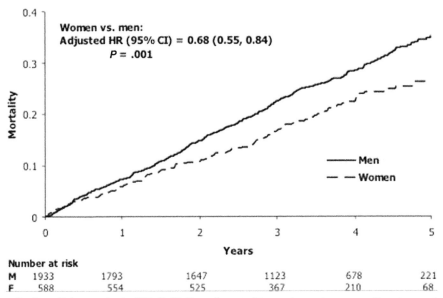

Fig. 3. Mortality benefit by gender in SCD-HeFT. Overall mortality was lower in women than in men in SCD-HeFT (P<.001). (*From* Russo AM, Poole JE, Mark DB, et al. Primary prevention with defibrillator therapy in women: results from the sudden cardiac death in heart failure trial. J Cardiovasc Electrophysiol 2008;19(7):722; with permission.)

enrollment or perhaps women may not meet enrollment criteria at the time of referral.

Other reasons for low percentage of enrolled women in ICD trials include gender differences in the prevalence of coronary artery disease (CAD) and inducibility of ventricular arrhythmias necessary to be eligible for enrollment in MUSTT, MADIT, and MADIT-II trials. Additionally, clinical trial enrollment may be skewed by the ages of participants; randomized trials that exclude subjects over a certain age are biased against women because women are known to have later onset and recognition of cardiovascular disease.[4,5]

Gender Differences in Implantable Cardioverter-Defibrillator Therapy

Gender differences exist in the incidence of potentially lethal arrhythmias and ICD shock therapy.

Women with established CAD with ICDs have lower rates of arrhythmias and electrical storms.[25] Analysis of primary prevention trials has shown that women have similar[10,26] or lower incidence[23,25,27,28] of appropriate ICD therapy in comparison to men. Literature demonstrates a linear relationship between the occurrence of shocks and adverse outcomes; as a result, male recipients of appropriate ICD therapy are a distinctive subgroup at higher risk for mortality.[26,29]

A review that included patients with ICM showed 18% higher incidence of sustained VT/VF requiring ICD therapy in men compared with women who received an ICD for primary prevention,[25] attributed to the higher frequency of myocardial scarring in men. Women were less likely than men to receive appropriate ICD shock or appropriate therapy via shock or ATP.[28]

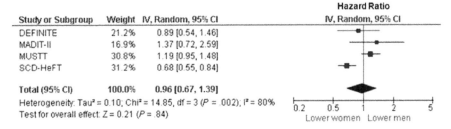

Fig. 4. Overall mortality benefit in primary prevention ICD trials. The Forest plot demonstrates the adjusted hazard ratio of overall mortality of women compared to men in each study and the overall adjusted hazard ratio. DF, degree of freedom; IV, Independent variable. (*From* Santangeli P, Pelargonio G, Dello Russo A, et al. Gender differences in clinical outcome and primary prevention defibrillator benefit in patients with severe left ventricular dysfunction: a systematic review and meta-analysis. Heart Rhythm 2010;7(7):879; with permission.)

ICD survival benefit among men

Study or Subgroup	Weight	IV, Random, 95% CI
SCD-HeFT	51.0%	0.71 [0.57, 0.88]
MADIT-II	23.5%	0.66 [0.48, 0.90]
DEFINITE	6.6%	0.49 [0.27, 0.88]
COMPANION	18.8%	0.65 [0.46, 0.92]
Total (95% CI)	100.0%	0.67 [0.58, 0.78]

Heterogeneity: Tau² = 0.00; Chi² = 1.40, df = 3 (P = .70); I² = 0%
Test for overall effect: Z = 5.17 (P < .00001)

Hazard Ratio
IV, Random, 95% CI

0.01   0.1   1   10   100
Favors ICD   Favors Placebo

ICD survival benefit among women

Study or Subgroup	Weight	IV, Random, 95% CI
SCD-HeFT	44.3%	0.90 [0.57, 1.43]
MADIT-II	18.9%	0.57 [0.28, 1.15]
DEFINITE	14.1%	1.14 [0.50, 2.58]
COMPANION	22.8%	0.59 [0.31, 1.12]
Total (95% CI)	100.0%	0.78 [0.57, 1.05]

Heterogeneity: Tau² = 0.00; Chi² = 2.69, df = 3 (P = .44); I² = 0%
Test for overall effect: Z = 1.63 (P = .10)

Hazard Ratio
IV, Random, 95% CI

0.01   0.1   1   10   100
Favors ICD   Favors Placebo

Fig. 5. ICD survival benefit among men and women in primary prevention ICD trials. The forest plots show the hazard ratio of survival benefit associated with ICD use in women and in men in each study and the overall hazard ratio. DF, degree of freedom; IV, Independent variable. (*From* Santangeli P, Pelargonio G, Dello Russo A, et al. Gender differences in clinical outcome and primary prevention defibrillator benefit in patients with severe left ventricular dysfunction: a systematic review and meta-analysis. Heart Rhythm 2010;7(7):880; with permission.)

Similarly, multiple studies and a meta-analysis also found a lower incidence of appropriate ICD therapy among women compared with men (**Fig. 6**).[12,23] In contrast, analysis of SCD-HeFT showed no significant difference in appropriate shock therapy among women and men.[26]

Gender Differences in Implantable Cardioverter-Defibrillator Complications

Several studies demonstrated that women were more likely to have both early and late procedural complications related to ICD implantation than men.[9,13,28,30,31] Device-related complications

were higher in women; specifically, women had increased rates of cardiac tamponade, hematoma requiring transfusion or evacuation, pneumothorax requiring chest tube, and 90-day mechanical complications requiring revision compared with men.[31] Although this finding is not well understood, it has been postulated that higher risk of perforation could be related to a thinner right ventricle and a higher incidence of pneumothorax could be related to smaller sized veins in women. Alternatively, women may receive ICDs at later stages of cardiac disease and have more advanced comorbidities, perhaps predisposing them to higher complication rates. Further analysis is required

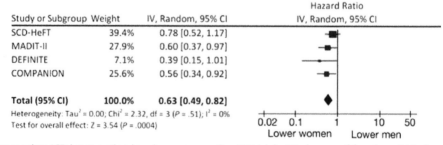

Study or Subgroup	Weight	IV, Random, 95% CI
SCD-HeFT	39.4%	0.78 [0.52, 1.17]
MADIT-II	27.9%	0.60 [0.37, 0.97]
DEFINITE	7.1%	0.39 [0.15, 1.01]
COMPANION	25.6%	0.56 [0.34, 0.92]
Total (95% CI)	100.0%	0.63 [0.49, 0.82]

Heterogeneity: Tau² = 0.00; Chi² = 2.32, df = 3 (P = .51); I² = 0%
Test for overall effect: Z = 3.54 (P = .0004)

Hazard Ratio
IV, Random, 95% CI

0.02   0.1   1   10   50
Lower women   Lower men

Fig. 6. Appropriate ICD intervention in primary prevention ICD trials. DF, degree of freedom; IV, Independent variable. The forest plot shows the adjusted hazard ratio of appropriate ICD intervention in women compared with men in each study and the overall adjusted hazard ratio. (*From* Santangeli P, Pelargonio G, Dello Russo A, et al. Gender differences in clinical outcome and primary prevention defibrillator benefit in patients with severe left ventricular dysfunction: a systematic review and meta-analysis. Heart Rhythm 2010;7(7):879; with permission.)

and is paramount to improving understanding of these gender differences.

Gender-Related Disparities

Although the use of ICDs has been shown to improve mortality, women are significantly less likely than men to receive this therapy for both primary and secondary prevention of SCD.[27,32] In a study comprising more than 132,000 patients with ischemic cardiomyopathy who were potential candidates for ICD therapy, men were more likely to receive an ICD than women.[33] In another large Medicare study comprising both patients in a primary and secondary prevention cohort, men were more likely to receive ICDs in both groups.[32] Similarly, a review reported that women were still 27% less likely to receive ICD for potentially lethal ventricular arrhythmias.[12]

Several potential reasons may explain this gender disparity in ICD receipt. It is possible that women were not referred due to advanced age with greater comorbidities, or women may be inaccurately perceived as low risk for SCD; alternatively, they may be declining referral for ICD placement.[34] It is also possible that provider bias may lead to under-referral of women.

An analysis of the GWTG-HF program examined 21,059 hospitalized HF patients and rates of ICD counseling among eligible patients. Up to 4 of 5 patients eligible for ICD did not receive counseling. Women were less frequently counseled than men; however, when appropriately counseled, women and men were equally as likely to receive an ICD.[35] Other plausible explanations for not undergoing ICD implantation included suboptimal communication between physician and patient, patient preference, and fragmented medical care, causing inadequate follow-up or specific contraindications not previously outlined.

Several studies have evaluated whether the disparities in ICD use have improved over time with counseling and after targeted interventions were applied. Among hospitals participating in GWTG-HF, overall rates of ICD implantation improved from 30% to 42% from 2005 to 2007. A significant increase in ICD therapy was observed over time in women, men, blacks and whites. Racial disparities in ICD use were no longer present by the end of the study period; however, gender differences persisted.[36] The IMPROVE-HF study introduced a program that provided educational materials and clinical decision-making support tools to health care providers. At the end of 2 years, the rate of ICD use increased from 49% to 79% in both men and women.[37] To continue improving ICD referral and placement, specific efforts are needed in both the hospital and clinic settings for recognition of eligible patients and appropriate counseling as well as time-sensitive follow-up of targeted patients.

Summary

Through recent decades, ICDs have become the mainstay of treatment of the primary and secondary prevention of SCD. Randomized trials have demonstrated that ICDs reduce mortality. Unfortunately, women were under-represented in these landmark trials and, as a result, trials were underpowered to detect significant differences by gender. Although gender differences may exist in baseline characteristics at enrollment and in mortality benefit, ICD shocks, and complication rates, current guidelines for ICD implantation do not support differential use by gender. Further research is necessary to better understand potential reasons for gender differences, with an emphasis on enrolling a higher proportion of women in future trials to help bridge knowledge gaps.

CARDIAC RESYNCHRONIZATION THERAPY
Dyssynchrony

Many changes are known to occur in a failing myocardium, including electrical dyssynchrony, mechanical dyssynchrony and cardiac remodeling. Approximately one-third of patients with NYHA class III/IV HF and systolic dysfunction experience mechanical dyssynchrony.[38] The aim of cardiac resynchronization therapy (CRT) is to restore mechanical synchrony by providing a more physiologic pattern of depolarization.

Gender Differences in Cardiac Resynchronization Therapy Outcomes

Several landmark trials, including MIRACLE-ICD, COMPANION, CARE-HF, MADIT-CRT and RAFT, demonstrated that CRT improved outcomes in patients with symptomatic HF with reduced ejection fraction and prolonged QRS duration.[39–43] These improved outcomes were not limited to mortality benefit but also included improved quality of life, decreased rates of hospitalization, and improved HF symptoms. Although these trials enrolled low numbers of women constituting only 17% to 33% of the study population, greater benefit of CRT was demonstrated among women compared with men.[44–48] **Table 4** summarizes the major CRT trials.

In the MIRACLE trial, women but not men receiving CRT were more likely to be event-free from first HF hospitalization or death compared with the control group.[39,45] In the MADIT-CRT trial, CRT-D therapy was shown to have greater effect

Table 4
Summary of cardiac resynchronization therapy trials

Study (Year)	Patients Enrolled = n (%)	Inclusion Criteria	Treatment Arms	Outcomes
MIRACLE-ICD (2003)	Men: 283 (77%) Women: 86 (23%)	NYHA II, LVEF ≤35%, QRS ≥130 ms	CRT-D vs ICD only	• CRT-ICD improved quality of life ($P = .02$), increased peak oxygen consumption ($P = .04$), increased treadmill exercise duration ($P<.001$) and improved functional class ($P = .007$)
COMPANION (2004)	Men: 1025 (67%) Women: 495 (33%)	NYHA III–IV, LVEF ≤35%, QRS >120 ms	OMT vs OMT + CRT-P vs OMT + CRT-D	• CRT-P and CRT-D ↓ risk of death or hospitalization for HF by 34% and 40% compared with medical therapy alone ($P<.002$, $P<.001$) • Death from any cause ↓ 24% in CRT-P ($P = .059$) and by 36% in CRT-D ($P = .003$) compared with medical therapy alone • NYHA class, 6-min distance walk test and quality of life improved in both CRT groups vs medical therapy alone ($0 < 0.001$)
CARE-HF (2005)	Men: 597 (73%) Women: 495 (27%)	NYHA III–IV, LVEF ≤35%, QRS >120 ms	OMT vs OMT + CRT	• Death/unplanned hospitalization for CV event ↓ 16% ($P<.001$) • 10% ↓ death from any cause in CRT group ($P<.01$) • 15% ↓ in hospitalizations for worsening HF, increased LVEF, and improved quality of life in CRT group ($P<.01$)

Trial	Sex distribution	Criteria	Comparison	Outcomes
MADIT-CRT (2009)	Men: 1367 (75%) Women: 453 (25%)	NYHA I–II, LVEF ≤30%, QRS ≥130 ms	CRT-D vs ICD alone	• 41% ↓ in risk of HF events (HR 0.59, 95% CI 0.47–0.74, $P<.001$) in CRT group
RAFT (2010)	Men: 1490 (83%) Women: 308 (17%)	NYHA II–III, LVEF ≤30%, QRS ≥120 ms	CRT vs ICD alone	• 25% RRR in death from any cause (HR 0.75; 95% CI, 0.62–0.91; $P = .003$) • 24% RRR in death from CV cause (HR 0.76; 95% CI, 0.6–0.96; $P = .02$) • 32% RRR in hospitalization for HF (HR 0.68; 95% CI, 0.56–0.83; $P<.001$)

Abbreviations: CARE-HF, Cardiac Resynchronization-Heart Failure; COMPANION, Comparison of Medical Therapy, Pacing, and Defibrillation in Heart Failure; CRT-D, cardiac resynchronization therapy defibrillator; CRT-P, cardiac resynchronization therapy pacemaker; HR, hazard ratio; MADIT-CRT, Multicenter Automatic Defibrillator Implantation Trial-CRT; MIRACLE-ICD, Multicenter InSync Randomized Clinical Evaluation (MIRACLE)-ICD; OMT, optimal medical therapy; RAFT, Resynchronization in Ambulatory Heart Failure Trial; RRR, relative risk reduction.

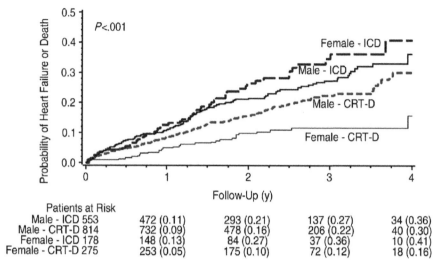

Patients at Risk

Male - ICD 553	472 (0.11)	293 (0.21)	137 (0.27)	34 (0.36)
Male - CRT-D 814	732 (0.09)	478 (0.16)	206 (0.22)	40 (0.30)
Female - ICD 178	148 (0.13)	84 (0.27)	37 (0.36)	10 (0.41)
Female - CRT-D 275	253 (0.05)	175 (0.10)	72 (0.12)	18 (0.16)

Fig. 7. Probability of HF or death stratified by gender and ICD versus CRT-D therapy. The curves reflect the probability of HF or death in women and men with ICDs or CRT-D devices. Women who received CRT-D therapy had the best outcomes. (*From* Arshad A, Moss AJ, Foster E, et al. Cardiac resynchronization therapy is more effective in women than in men: the MADIT-CRT (Multicenter Automatic Defibrillator Implantation Trial with Cardiac Resynchronization Therapy) trial. J Am Coll Cardiol 2011;57(7):816; with permission.)

in women than in men.[42] In addition to gender, etiology of heart disease significantly influenced risk for VT/VF or death. Women with ischemic heart disease and women with LBBB who received CRT-D had the lowest incidence of VT/VF or death compared with men.[49]

In contrast to ICD trials, CRT device trials have consistently demonstrated lower all-cause mortality in women than in men receiving CRT. A meta-analysis of 3 major CRT versus CRT-D trials (MADIT-CRT, RAFT, and REVERSE) found 76% reduction in mortality among women with CRT without similar benefit in men.[50] Similarly, a 69% reduction in HF or death, 72% reduction in all-cause mortality, and 82% and 78% reductions in mortality in those with QRS greater than 150 ms with LBBB was found in women (**Fig. 7**).[44]

Several studies have evaluated gender differences in HF hospitalizations. A closer analysis of the MIRACLE study found that women with CRT had a longer time to first HF hospitalization or death.[45] This information was consistent with findings from COMPANION, CARE-HF, and MADIT-CRT trials that also showed significant reduction in HF or death in CRT-D arms among women.[40–42]

Reasons for Gender Differences in Cardiac Resynchronization Therapy Trials

Several CRT studies, including REVERSE, MADIT-CRT and RAFT, suggested that women have a more favorable response to CRT compared with men.[42,43,51] In response to this finding, potential mechanisms for better CRT outcomes among

women were investigated: women had better reverse modeling leading to greater reductions in left ventricular (LV) volumes, better atrioventricular optimization, greater reductions in LV end-systolic volumes and a greater percentage of biventricular pacing in comparison to men, despite similar baseline characteristics at enrollment.[46]

Among the CRT trials, women were more likely to have a nonischemic etiology of cardiomyopathy. In addition, they were more likely to have a smaller overall scar burden on cardiac MRI compared with men in the ICD group. In the CRT group, there was a higher prevalence of NICM contributing to a smaller scar size in women. It was concluded that although increased myocardial scar burden was associated with more appropriate ICD shocks in men, it also led to decreased responsiveness to CRT, possibly contributing to the observed gender differences in device benefit.[52]

Men were more likely to have atrial fibrillation and renal dysfunction compared with women,[44] 2 factors that have been associated with poorer prognosis and higher risk of death in the MADIT-II population.[53] Men were also more likely to have right bundle branch block, which has been associated with poorer outcomes with CRT.[54] Overall, men had more risk factors associated with poorer CRT response, which could explain why women experienced better outcomes.

Healthy women have shorter QRS complexes in comparison to men.[55] As a result, for women to meet CRT criteria, they need to have more severe intracardiac conduction abnormalities. With shorter QRS durations at baseline, a similar degree

Cardiac Resynchronization Therapy in Patients With Systolic Heart Failure

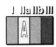

CRT is indicated for patients who have left ventricular ejection fraction (LVEF) less than or equal to 35%, sinus rhythm, LBBB with a QRS duration greater than or equal to 150 ms, and NYHA class II, III, or ambulatory IV symptoms on GDMT. *(Level of Evidence: A for NYHA class III/IV; Level of Evidence: B for NYHA class II).*

CRT can be useful for patients who have LVEF less than or equal to 35%, sinus rhythm, LBBB with a QRS duration 120 to 149 ms, and NYHA class II, III, or ambulatory IV symptoms on GDMT.

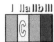

CRT can be useful for patients who have LVEF less than or equal to 35%, sinus rhythm, a non-LBBB pattern with a QRS duration greater than or equal to 150 ms, and NYHA class III/ambulatory class IV symptoms on GDMT.

CRT can be useful in patients with atrial fibrillation and LVEF less than or equal to 35% on GDMT if a) the patient requires ventricular pacing or otherwise meets CRT criteria and b) AV nodal ablation or pharmacologic rate control will allow near 100% ventricular pacing with CRT.

CRT can be useful for patients on GDMT who have LVEF less than or equal to 35% and are undergoing new or replacement device placement with anticipated requirement for significant (>40%) ventricular pacing.

CRT may be considered for patients who have LVEF less than or equal to 30%, ischemic etiology of heart failure, sinus rhythm, LBBB with a QRS duration of greater than or equal to 150 ms, and NYHA class I symptoms on GDMT.

CRT may be considered for patients who have LVEF less than or equal to 35%, sinus rhythm, a non-LBBB pattern with QRS duration 120 to 149 ms, and NYHA class III/ambulatory class IV on GDMT.

CRT may be considered for patients who have LVEF less than or equal to 35%, sinus rhythm, a non-LBBB pattern with a QRS duration greater than or equal to 150 ms, and NYHA class II symptoms on GDMT.

CRT is not recommended for patients with NYHA class I or II symptoms and non-LBBB pattern with QRS duration less than 150 ms.

CRT is not indicated for patients whose comorbidities and/or frailty limit survival with good functional capacity to less than 1 y.

Fig. 8. ACCF/AHA/HRS CRT 2012 indications. Indications for CRT are illustrated in the 2012 focused update of the device-based therapy practice guidelines. (*Data from* Tracy CM, Epstein AE, Darbar D, et al. 2012 ACCF/AHA/HRS focused update incorporated into the ACCF/AHA/HRS 2008 guidelines for device-based therapy of cardiac rhythm abnormalities: a report of the American College of Cardiology Foundation/American Heart Association Task Force on Practice Guidelines and the Heart Rhythm Society. J Am Coll Cardiol 2013;61(3):e25.)

of QRS prolongation in women represents a greater deviation from normal and may result in greater dyssynchrony.

Further mechanisms for improved response to CRT in women were studied. Combined patient data from the RAFT, REVERSE, and MADIT-CRT trials was examined and found that among patients with LBBB with CRT-D, mortality was lower in women compared with men and that longer QRS duration of LBBB is associated with better outcomes, specifically among women.[56,57] This further solidified the hypothesis that the greater benefit of CRT may be seen with a shorter absolute QRS duration in women.

It is presumed that smaller cardiac size and mass are reasons why women may have better

LV reverse remodeling and shorter QRS duration on average[58,59] and, thus, one of the reasons why women seem to benefit more from CRT. Current clinical guidelines have the same recommendations for CRT therapy in both women and men (**Fig. 8**).[60] Overall, women had a higher response rate than men at a shorter QRS duration.[61] Given the evidence supporting better outcomes of CRT in women with shorter QRS durations compared with men, future guidelines may eventually reflect recommendations tailored by gender.

Under-Representation of Women in Cardiac Resynchronization Therapy Trials and Device Referral Disparities

In comparison to the ICD trials, there was a slightly higher percentage of women enrolled (17%–33%) in CRT trials; however, under-representation of women was evident in these studies as well (see **Table 4**). Despite a clear mortality benefit, decrease in hospitalization for HF and improvement in reverse modeling among women receiving CRT, eligible women are still less likely than men to receive this therapy.

Several explanations may help explain this gender difference and are similar to theories for ICD placement. Advanced age with greater comorbidities, referral bias, family responsibilities, and potential fear of fetal consequences for women of child-bearing age are possible reasons why women may be less likely to receive CRT. Women have higher rates of HFpEF but experience more symptomatic HF symptoms and have worse NYHA class.[59] Because CRT trials and guidelines require an LVEF less than or equal to 35%, fewer women with HF may meet inclusion criteria based on LV systolic function compared with men. There is also evidence that women are treated less aggressively for heart disease and are less likely to receive guideline-recommended treatments, suggesting potential referral bias.[62,63]

After implementation of the AHA GWTG-HF quality initiative program, increased use of CRT was noted. HF patients from this quality-improvement initiative were examined and, despite improvement in the numbers of CRT devices implanted, women were less likely to receive this therapy and this difference increased over time despite greater mortality risk reduction.[64] With the application of a performance improvement program, the use of CRT increased from 37% to 66% in men and women over 2 years.[65]

Summary

Clinical trials demonstrate a significant improvement in mortality, reduced hospitalization rates and improved symptoms among both women and men who receive CRT. The studies discussed previously and meta-analyses demonstrate that response to CRT differs by gender. Guideline recommendations remain gender neutral for implantation of CRT, although studies suggest women benefit more than men at shorter QRS duration. Unfortunately, women are under-represented in CRT trials, as was the case with ICD trials. Further research is needed in this area to address these findings and evaluate potential mechanisms for gender differences. The apparent benefit of CRT at a shorter QRS duration in women suggests that a larger cohort of women may potentially benefit if CRT guidelines are expanded. In addition, overall enrollment of women in future clinical trials needs to be more robust to ensure that results are applicable to both genders.

REFERENCES

1. Centers for Disease Control and Prevention (CDC). State-specific mortality from sudden cardiac death–United States, 1999. MMWR Morb Mortal Wkly Rep 2002;51(6):123–6.
2. Kim C, Fahrenbruch CE, Cobb LA, et al. Out-of-hospital cardiac arrest in men and women. Circulation 2001;104(22):2699–703.
3. Albert CM, Chae CU, Grodstein F, et al. Prospective study of sudden cardiac death among women in the United States. Circulation 2003;107(16):2096–101.
4. Deo R, Albert CM. Epidemiology and genetics of sudden cardiac death. Circulation 2012;125(4): 620–37.
5. Chugh SS, Uy-Evanado A, Teodorescu C, et al. Women have a lower prevalence of structural heart disease as a precursor to sudden cardiac arrest: the Ore-SUDS (Oregon Sudden Unexpected Death Study). J Am Coll Cardiol 2009; 54(22):2006–11.
6. Bosson N, Kaji AH, Fang A, et al. Sex differences in survival from out-of-hospital cardiac arrest in the era of regionalized systems and advanced post-resuscitation care. J Am Heart Assoc 2016;5(9). https://doi.org/10.1161/JAHA.116.004131.
7. Bougouin W, Mustafic H, Marijon E, et al. Gender and survival after sudden cardiac arrest: a systematic review and meta-analysis. Resuscitation 2015; 94:55–60.
8. Al-Khatib SM, Stevenson WG, Ackerman MJ, et al. 2017 AHA/ACC/HRS guideline for management of patients with ventricular arrhythmias and the prevention of sudden cardiac death: a report of the American College of Cardiology/American Heart Association Task Force on Clinical Practice Guidelines and the Heart Rhythm Society. Circulation 2017. https://doi.org/10.1161/CIR.0000000000000549.

9. Peterson PN, Daugherty SL, Wang Y, et al. Gender differences in procedure-related adverse events in patients receiving implantable cardioverter-defibrillator therapy. Circulation 2009;119(8):1078–84.

10. Russo AM, Stamato NJ, Lehmann MH, et al. Influence of gender on arrhythmia characteristics and outcome in the Multicenter UnSustained Tachycardia Trial. J Cardiovasc Electrophysiol 2004;15(9):993–8.

11. Moss AJ, Zareba W, Hall WJ, et al. Prophylactic implantation of a defibrillator in patients with myocardial infarction and reduced ejection fraction. N Engl J Med 2002;346(12):877–83.

12. Santangeli P, Pelargonio G, Dello Russo A, et al. Gender differences in clinical outcome and primary prevention defibrillator benefit in patients with severe left ventricular dysfunction: a systematic review and meta-analysis. Heart Rhythm 2010;7(7):876–82.

13. Albert CM, Quigg R, Saba S, et al. Sex differences in outcome after implantable cardioverter defibrillator implantation in nonischemic cardiomyopathy. Am Heart J 2008;156(2):367–72.

14. Kadish A, Dyer A, Daubert JP, et al. Prophylactic defibrillator implantation in patients with nonischemic dilated cardiomyopathy. N Engl J Med 2004; 350(21):2151–8.

15. Bardy GH, Lee KL, Mark DB, et al. Amiodarone or an implantable cardioverter–defibrillator for congestive heart failure. N Engl J Med 2005;352(3):225–37.

16. Russo AM, Poole JE, Mark DB, et al. Primary prevention with defibrillator therapy in women: results from the sudden cardiac death in heart failure trial. J Cardiovasc Electrophysiol 2008;19(7):720–4.

17. Buxton AE, Lee KL, Fisher JD, et al. A randomized study of the prevention of sudden death in patients with coronary artery disease. N Engl J Med 1999; 341(25):1882–90.

18. Zeitler EP, Hellkamp AS, Schulte PJ, et al. Comparative effectiveness of implantable cardioverter defibrillators for primary prevention in women. Circ Heart Fail 2016;9(1):e002630.

19. Henyan NN, White CM, Gillespie EL, et al. The impact of gender on survival amongst patients with implantable cardioverter defibrillators for primary prevention against sudden cardiac death. J Intern Med 2006;260(5):467–73.

20. Antiarrhythmics Versus Implantable Defibrillators (AVID) Investigators. A comparison of antiarrhythmic-drug therapy with implantable defibrillators in patients resuscitated from near-fatal ventricular arrhythmias. N Engl J Med 1997;337(22):1576–84.

21. Kuck KH, Cappato R, Siebels J, et al. Randomized comparison of antiarrhythmic drug therapy with implantable defibrillators in patients resuscitated from cardiac arrest: the Cardiac Arrest Study Hamburg (CASH). Circulation 2000;102(7):748–54.

22. Connolly SJ, Gent M, Roberts RS, et al. Canadian implantable defibrillator study (CIDS): a randomized trial of the implantable cardioverter defibrillator against amiodarone. Circulation 2000;101(11):1297–302.

23. Ghanbari H, Dalloul G, Hasan R, et al. Effectiveness of implantable cardioverter-defibrillators for the primary prevention of sudden cardiac death in women with advanced heart failure: a meta-analysis of randomized controlled trials. Arch Intern Med 2009; 169(16):1500–6.

24. Melloni C, Berger JS, Wang TY, et al. Representation of women in randomized clinical trials of cardiovascular disease prevention. Circ Cardiovasc Qual Outcomes 2010;3(2):135–42.

25. Lampert R, McPherson CA, Clancy JF, et al. Gender differences in ventricular arrhythmia recurrence in patients with coronary artery disease and implantable cardioverter-defibrillators. J Am Coll Cardiol 2004;43(12):2293–9.

26. Poole JE, Johnson GW, Hellkamp AS, et al. Prognostic importance of defibrillator shocks in patients with heart failure. N Engl J Med 2008;359(10): 1009–17.

27. Seegers J, Conen D, Jung K, et al. Sex difference in appropriate shocks but not mortality during long-term follow-up in patients with implantable cardioverter-defibrillators. Europace 2016;18(8):1194–202.

28. MacFadden DR, Crystal E, Krahn AD, et al. Sex differences in implantable cardioverter-defibrillator outcomes: findings from a prospective defibrillator database. Ann Intern Med 2012;156(3):195–203.

29. Moss AJ, Greenberg H, Case RB, et al. Long-term clinical course of patients after termination of ventricular tachyarrhythmia by an implanted defibrillator. Circulation 2004;110(25):3760–5.

30. Masoudi FA, Go AS, Magid DJ, et al. Age and sex differences in long-term outcomes following implantable cardioverter-defibrillator placement in contemporary clinical practice: findings from the cardiovascular research network. J Am Heart Assoc 2015;4(6). https://doi.org/10.1161/JAHA.115.002005.

31. Russo AM, Daugherty SL, Masoudi FA, et al. Gender and outcomes after primary prevention implantable cardioverter-defibrillator implantation: findings from the National Cardiovascular Data Registry (NCDR). Am Heart J 2015;170(2):330–8.

32. Curtis LH, Al-Khatib SM, Shea AM, et al. Sex differences in the use of implantable cardioverter-defibrillators for primary and secondary prevention of sudden cardiac death. JAMA 2007;298(13): 1517–24.

33. Gauri AJ, Davis A, Hong T, et al. Disparities in the use of primary prevention and defibrillator therapy among blacks and women. Am J Med 2006; 119(2):167.e17–21.

34. Staniforth AD, Sporton SC, Robinson NM, et al. Is there a sex bias in implantable cardioverter-defibrillator referral and prescription? Heart 2004; 90(8):937–8.

35. Hess PL, Hernandez AF, Bhatt DL, et al. Sex and race/ethnicity differences in implantable cardioverter-defibrillator counseling and use among patients hospitalized with heart failure: findings from the get with the guidelines-heart failure program. Circulation 2016. https://doi.org/10.1161/CIRCULATIONAHA.115.021048.

36. Al-Khatib SM, Hellkamp AS, Hernandez AF, et al. Trends in use of implantable cardioverter-defibrillator therapy among patients hospitalized for heart failure: have the previously observed sex and racial disparities changed over time? Circulation 2012;125(9):1094–101.

37. Walsh MN, Yancy CW, Albert NM, et al. Equitable improvement for women and men in the use of guideline-recommended therapies for heart failure: findings from IMPROVE HF. J Card Fail 2010;16(12):940–9.

38. McAlister FA, Ezekowitz J, Hooton N, et al. Cardiac resynchronization therapy for patients with left ventricular systolic dysfunction: a systematic review. JAMA 2007;297(22):2502–14.

39. Young JB, Abraham WT, Smith AL, et al. Combined cardiac resynchronization and implantable cardioversion defibrillation in advanced chronic heart failure: the MIRACLE ICD Trial. JAMA 2003;289(20):2685–94.

40. Bristow MR, Saxon LA, Boehmer J, et al. Cardiac-resynchronization therapy with or without an implantable defibrillator in advanced chronic heart failure. N Engl J Med 2004;350(21):2140–50.

41. Cleland JGF, Daubert J-C, Erdmann E, et al. The effect of cardiac resynchronization on morbidity and mortality in heart failure. N Engl J Med 2005;352(15):1539–49.

42. Moss AJ, Hall WJ, Cannom DS, et al. Cardiac-resynchronization therapy for the prevention of heart-failure events. N Engl J Med 2009;361(14):1329–38.

43. Tang ASL, Wells GA, Talajic M, et al. Cardiac-resynchronization therapy for mild-to-moderate heart failure. N Engl J Med 2010;363(25):2385–95.

44. Arshad A, Moss AJ, Foster E, et al. Cardiac resynchronization therapy is more effective in women than in men: the MADIT-CRT (Multicenter Automatic Defibrillator Implantation Trial with Cardiac Resynchronization Therapy) trial. J Am Coll Cardiol 2011;57(7):813–20.

45. Woo GW, Petersen-Stejskal S, Johnson JW, et al. Ventricular reverse remodeling and 6-month outcomes in patients receiving cardiac resynchronization therapy: analysis of the MIRACLE study. J Interv Card Electrophysiol 2005;12(2):107–13.

46. Cheng A, Gold MR, Waggoner AD, et al. Potential mechanisms underlying the effect of gender on response to cardiac resynchronization therapy: insights from the SMART-AV multicenter trial. Heart Rhythm 2012;9(5):736–41.

47. Herz ND, Engeda J, Zusterzeel R, et al. Sex differences in device therapy for heart failure: utilization, outcomes, and adverse events. J Womens Health 2015;24(4):261–71.

48. Leyva F, Foley PWX, Chalil S, et al. Female gender is associated with a better outcome after cardiac resynchronization therapy. Pacing Clin Electrophysiol 2011;34(1):82–8.

49. Tompkins CM, Kutyifa V, Arshad A, et al. Sex differences in device therapies for ventricular arrhythmias or death in the multicenter automatic defibrillator implantation trial with cardiac resynchronization therapy (MADIT-CRT) trial. J Cardiovasc Electrophysiol 2015;26(8):862–71.

50. Zusterzeel R, Selzman KA, Sanders WE, et al. Cardiac resynchronization therapy in women: US Food and Drug Administration meta-analysis of patient-level data. JAMA Intern Med 2014;174(8):1340–8.

51. Linde C, Abraham WT, Gold MR, et al. Randomized trial of cardiac resynchronization in mildly symptomatic heart failure patients and in asymptomatic patients with left ventricular dysfunction and previous heart failure symptoms. J Am Coll Cardiol 2008;52(23):1834–43.

52. Loring Z, Strauss DG, Gerstenblith G, et al. Cardiac MRI scar patterns differ by sex in an implantable cardioverter-defibrillator and cardiac resynchronization therapy cohort. Heart Rhythm 2013;10(5):659–65.

53. Goldenberg I, Vyas AK, Hall WJ, et al. Risk stratification for primary implantation of a cardioverter-defibrillator in patients with ischemic left ventricular dysfunction. J Am Coll Cardiol 2008;51(3):288–96.

54. Gervais R, Leclercq C, Shankar A, et al. Surface electrocardiogram to predict outcome in candidates for cardiac resynchronization therapy: a subanalysis of the CARE-HF trial. Eur J Heart Fail 2009;11(7):699–705.

55. Macfarlane PW, McLaughlin SC, Devine B, et al. Effects of age, sex, and race on ECG interval measurements. J Electrocardiol 1994;27(Suppl):14–9.

56. Zusterzeel R, Curtis JP, Caños DA, et al. Sex-specific mortality risk by QRS morphology and duration in patients receiving CRT: results from the NCDR. J Am Coll Cardiol 2014;64(9):887–94.

57. Zusterzeel R, Spatz ES, Curtis JP, et al. Cardiac resynchronization therapy in women versus men: observational comparative effectiveness study from the national cardiovascular data registry. Circ Cardiovasc Qual Outcomes 2015. https://doi.org/10.1161/CIRCOUTCOMES.114.001548.

58. Hnatkova K, Smetana P, Toman O, et al. Sex and race differences in QRS duration. Europace 2016;18(12):1842–9.

59. Yin F-H, Fan C-L, Guo Y-Y, et al. The impact of gender difference on clinical and echocardiographic outcomes in patients with heart failure after

cardiac resynchronization therapy: a systematic review and meta-analysis. PLoS ONE 2017;12(4). https://doi.org/10.1371/journal.pone.0176248.

60. Tracy CM, Epstein AE, Darbar D, et al. 2012 ACCF/AHA/HRS focused update incorporated into the ACCF/AHA/HRS 2008 guidelines for device-based therapy of cardiac rhythm abnormalities: a report of the American College of Cardiology Foundation/American Heart Association Task Force on Practice Guidelines and the Heart Rhythm Society. J Am Coll Cardiol 2013;61(3):e6–75.

61. Varma N, Manne M, Nguyen D, et al. Probability and magnitude of response to cardiac resynchronization therapy according to QRS duration and gender in nonischemic cardiomyopathy and LBBB. Heart Rhythm 2014;11(7):1139–47.

62. Lenzen MJ, Rosengren A, Scholte op Reimer WJM, et al. Management of patients with heart failure in clinical practice: differences between men and women. Heart 2008;94(3):e10.

63. Burstein JM, Yan R, Weller I, et al. Management of congestive heart failure: a gender gap may still exist. Observations from a contemporary cohort. BMC Cardiovasc Disord 2003;3(1):1.

64. Randolph TC, Hellkamp AS, Zeitler EP, et al. Utilization of cardiac resynchronization therapy in eligible patients hospitalized for heart failure and its association with patient outcomes. Am Heart J 2017;189: 48–58.

65. Fonarow GC, Albert NM, Curtis AB, et al. Improving evidence-based care for heart failure in outpatient cardiology practices: primary results of the Registry to Improve the Use of Evidence-Based Heart Failure Therapies in the Outpatient Setting (IMPROVE HF). Circulation 2010;122(6):585–96.

Heart Transplantation in Women

Ayesha Hasan, MD[a], Michelle M. Kittleson, MD, PhD[b],*

KEYWORDS

- Sensitization • Rejection • Survival • Quality of life

KEY POINTS

- Survival after heart transplantation is greater in women than in men, although women experience more depression and less satisfaction with health and functioning long term after transplant.
- Successful pregnancy after transplantation requires an early, well-planned multidisciplinary approach to all stages of pregnancy, from preconception counseling and assessment of a patient's graft function to immunosuppression to a delivery plan involving the entire care team, particularly in the scenario of peripartum graft dysfunction.
- Women are more likely to be sensitized, with preformed anti-human leukocyte antigens (HLA) antibodies related to prior pregnancies. Identification of potentially cytotoxic donor-specific anti-HLA antibodies prior to transplantation via complement-fixation assays and reduction with plasmapheresis/bortezomib and neutralization with eculizumab offer hope of heart transplantation for such highly sensitized candidates.

INTRODUCTION

Over the past 5 decades, heart transplantation has become an established therapy with greater quality of life and survival than can be expected from end-stage heart failure. Despite major advances in the treatment of end-stage heart disease, many patients with refractory heart failure, progressive angina, or uncontrolled ventricular arrhythmias cannot be stabilized with medical or interventional/surgical therapy and suffer significant morbidity and mortality.[1] For such patients, cardiac transplantation is widely accepted to improve quality and quantity of life.

Women comprise approximately half of all transplant recipients internationally[2] and offer specific challenges in management. Women have better survival but fare worse on certain health-related quality-of-life assessments. Pregnancy after transplantation is possible but needs to be carefully managed with regard to the effects of immunosuppression on the fetus and the hemodynamic effects of pregnancy on the transplanted heart. Women are also more likely to be sensitized, and the presence of preformed anti-HLA antibodies poses an increased risk of antibody-mediated rejection after transplantation.

This article focuses on the outcomes of women after transplantation, management strategies for pregnancy after heart transplantation, and recent advances in the approach to the sensitized heart transplant recipient.

POST-TRANSPLANT OUTCOMES

Survival

Survival after heart transplantation has steadily improved in the past 3 decades. In the 1980s, 1-year survival was 70% and the conditional half-life, the time at which 50% of patients who

Disclosure: The authors have nothing to disclose.
[a] Clinical Internal Medicine, Cardiac Transplant Program, Heart Failure Fellowship Program, Ohio State University Wexner Medical Center, 200 DHLRI, 473 West 12th Avenue, Columbus, OH 43220, USA; [b] Education in Heart Failure and Transplantation, Heart Failure Research, Smidt Heart Institute, Cedars-Sinai Medical Center, 8536 Wilshire Boulevard Suite 301, Los Angeles, CA 90211, USA
* Corresponding author.
E-mail address: michelle.kittleson@cshs.org

Heart Failure Clin 15 (2019) 127–135
https://doi.org/10.1016/j.hfc.2018.08.012
1551-7136/19/© 2018 Elsevier Inc. All rights reserved.

survived the first year are still alive, was 9.4 years. In the 2017 report from the International Society of Heart and Lung Transplantation (ISHLT) registry,[2] 1-year survival is approximately 90%, with a conditional half-life of more than 13 years. The mortality rate beyond 1 year after transplant has improved only marginally for patients who received allografts after 1992, and there has been no statistically significant improvement in the past 2 decades. This stable annual mortality rate of approximately 3% to 4% is higher than that of the general population and likely exists because the processes responsible for long-term mortality, including cardiac allograft vasculopathy and malignancy, remain a challenge of detection and treatment.

Female heart transplant recipients have better survival than their male counterparts. Female heart transplant recipients have a median survival of 11.5 years compared with 10.5 years in men. Conditional half-life is also higher in women, 14.4 years versus 13.0 years in men.[2] The reason for this is not clear and occurs despite the fact that women undergoing heart transplant are more likely to be sensitized (have preformed anti-HLA antibodies) than men.

An in-depth analysis of risk factors for survival at 1 year, 5 years, 10 years, 15 years, and 20 years after transplant is provided in the ISHLT registry report.[2] The strongest risk factors for 1-year mortality, associated with a 50% or more increase in the risk of 1-year mortality, are mainly related to technical issues and the underlying disease responsible for transplantation, including congenital cardiomyopathy versus nonischemic cardiomyopathy, prior transplant, pretransplant ventilatory support, or dialysis. Risk factors for 5-year and 10-year mortality, on the other hand, are most referable to immunologic issues and toxicity related to immunosuppression, including dialysis or infection after transplant, rejection during the first post-transplant year, and recipient history of diabetes and cancer.

Transplant era influences 20-year survival; those patients transplanted in 1995 have better 20-year survival than those transplanted in 1991.[2] Other factors affecting 20-year survival include etiology for transplantation, age, ischemic time, and center volume.[2]

Quality of Life

Not only do patients gain increased quantity of life after transplantation but also quality of life is improved. In the first years after heart transplant, approximately 75% of recipients report having a normal healthy lifestyle or only few disease symptoms, an additional 15% participate in normal activities with some difficulty, and less than 10% report a higher degree of limitations.[2]

Based on information from the ISHLT registry, many patients return to work after transplant. Among recipients aged 25 years old to 55 years old, approximately 50% were employed 5 years after transplantation.[2] On the basis of the functional data reviewed previously, it is apparent that additional recipients could return to the workplace; however, in the United States, the structure of disability benefits and health insurance considerations may represent a barrier to this process.

Although overall quality of life is good, and although women have better long-term survival after transplant than men, female heart transplant recipients have worse functional ability both early and later after heart transplantation[3,4] and more depression later after heart transplantation.[5] Gender was not related to work status[6] or overall satisfaction with health-related quality of life, although being female was related to less satisfaction with health and functioning long-term after transplant.[7] Although women reported more difficulty adhering to the transplant regimen, they demonstrated more actual adherence than men. Women reported using more negative coping styles but reported more satisfaction with social support.[8] Understanding the gender differences in health-related quality of life, coping styles, and coping resources is important because it may provide guidance in tailoring long-term care after heart transplantation.

PREGNANCY AFTER HEART TRANSPLANTATION

Pregnancy after transplantation is an important consideration in the current era of heart transplantation because many recipients are of, or survive to, childbearing age.[2] The first solid organ transplant pregnancy and delivery was reported in 1958 in a kidney recipient. Thirty years later, in 1988, a woman post–heart transplant had a successful delivery.[9] The National Transplantation Pregnancy Registry (NTPR) includes successful outcomes of pregnancy in thoracic organ transplant recipients.[10] Successful management requires a multidisciplinary approach addressing all stages of pregnancy: preconception counseling, optimal timing of pregnancy, immunosuppression management, monitoring for potential adverse maternal and fetal outcomes, postdelivery care, and monitoring for potential long-term maternal complications, such as rejection if sensitization develops.

Preconception Counseling

Preconception counseling should begin in the pretransplant period and review the risks to the mother and fetus, including rejection, infection, graft dysfunction, and teratogenic effects of immunosuppression.[11] HLA sensitization against paternal genes may occur. In one case, a mother with multiple prior episodes of acute cellular rejection in the first post-transplant year developed antibodies against paternal HLA after suffering a miscarriage and subsequently had antibody-mediated rejection 6 years after transplant.[12]

The etiology of the mother's cardiomyopathy must be taken into consideration because some cardiac diseases are hereditary. For example, congenital heart disease has a recurrence rate of up to 8% in offspring, and familial cardiomyopathies with a genetic basis exist.[13,14] Women with potentially inheritable conditions should undergo preconception genetic counseling. For women with pretransplant peripartum cardiomyopathy, the risk of rejection is higher within the first year after transplant and overall survival is reduced.[15] The risk of recurrence of peripartum cardiomyopathy after transplant, however, is uncertain. Most centers take a conservative approach and discourage pregnancy in such patients.

Assessing Clinical Status and Graft Function for Timing of Pregnancy

Hemodynamic changes occur early in pregnancy: a 30% to 50% increase in intravascular volume in the second trimester, a decline in systemic vascular resistance in the first/second trimesters, and a 10 beats-per-minute to 20 beats-per-minute rise in heart rate (**Fig. 1**).[16] If graft dysfunction or valvular disease limits cardiac output, the extra volume is poorly tolerated and results in heart failure. Labor also marks an additional increase in cardiac output; large volume shifts occur after delivery and can be heightened by the release of vena cava obstruction from a contracted uterus. The denervated heart responds to the demands of these changes in 2 ways: (1) increasing stroke volume through Frank-Starling mechanism due to the higher preload from the expanded intravascular volume and (2) increased heart rate and contractility from circulating catecholamines.

The American Society of Transplantation Consensus Conference on Reproductive Issues and Transplantation recommends the following considerations before pregnancy in any transplant recipient: no rejection in the past year, adequate and stable graft function, maintenance immunosuppression at stable dosing, and no acute infections that could harm the fetus.[17] The 2010 ISHLT guidelines for patient care recommend coronary evaluation within 6 months of pregnancy and biopsy/right heart catheterization before pregnancy

if indicated.[18] Comorbidities and baseline liver/renal function, including proteinuria, should be reviewed; vaccinations need to be up to date (influenza, pneumococcus, hepatitis B, and tetanus). Pregnancy should be discouraged in situations of persistent graft dysfunction and comorbidities, such as coronary allograft vasculopathy.

Regarding timing of conception, the general recommendation is to wait until after the first post-transplant year. Prenatal care includes frequent monitoring of blood pressure, urine culture, blood pressure, and for markers of pre-eclampsia.[17,18] Biopsy surveillance might be deferred during pregnancy or, when clinically indicated, performed with echocardiography instead of fluoroscopy or with appropriate lead shielding of the fetus.

Immunosuppression Management

The potential teratogenic effects of maintenance immunosuppression regimen must be reviewed prior to pregnancy. All immunosuppressive drugs enter the fetal circulation. Corticosteroids and calcineurin inhibitors (CNIs) are generally considered safe as Food and Drug Administration (FDA) category C, but the antimetabolite, mycophenolate mofetil (MMF) is FDA category D due to teratogenic effects.[11,18] MMF can cause external ear and other craniofacial deformities, such as cleft palate and lip, as well as first-trimester pregnancy loss.[19] Azathioprine (AZA) is also category D with reports of fetal malformation. Mammalian target of rapamycin (mTOR) inhibitors, sirolimus and everolimus, have few data, suggesting they only be used if other well-established drugs are contraindicated.[16] When used during pregnancy, mTOR inhibitors should be changed to CNIs if cesarean section is planned due to associated poor wound healing.[11]

ISHLT guidelines recommend continuing CNIs and corticosteroids but avoiding MMF.[18] Use of other drugs, such as AZA, may be used, based on the individual patient and risk/benefit profile. Drug levels require close monitoring during pregnancy due to changes in metabolism and circulating blood volume. For example, CNI levels tend to decrease due maternal cytochrome P450 3A4 activity.[16]

In the postpartum period, immunosuppression may need to be reduced if increased during pregnancy due to the transient higher metabolism rates; thus, drug levels still require close monitoring. Because immunosuppression drugs are secreted in breastmilk, the ISHLT recommends against breastfeeding because the effects on infants remain undetermined[18]; conversely, the

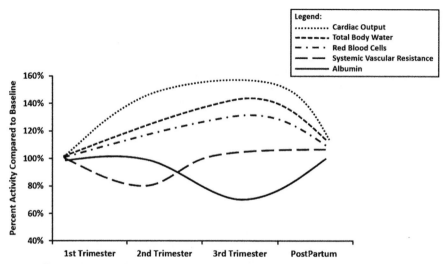

Fig. 1. Summary of hemodynamic changes during pregnancy. Cardiac output increases early in pregnancy, peaking in the second trimester and remaining at this level through delivery; it is driven by in an increase in stroke volume from the expansion in blood volume. The rise in total body water exceeds the rise in red blood cell production, leading to dilutional anemia in the mother. Systemic vascular resistance declines early in pregnancy due to progesterone levels, offsetting the volume expansion. Peripheral edema is related to the decline in albumin noted later in pregnancy but also influenced by the rise in total body water and the effect of fetal compression on the inferior vena cava. (*From* Casale JP, Doligalski CT. Pharmacologic considerations for solid organ transplant recipients who become pregnant. Pharmacotherapy 2016;36(9):975; with permission.)

American Society of Transplantation states it is not absolutely contraindicated for this reason.[17]

Adverse Maternal and Fetal Outcomes

The most common complication in the pregnant heart transplant recipient is hypertension. The NTPR reported hypertension in 43% and preeclampsia in 11% of pregnant heart transplant recipients.[20] Infection is another common complication (reported in 14%), and routine screening for urine infections is recommended[20] CMV seroconversion or reactivation should be monitored during pregnancy due to the perinatal risk of maternal CMV viremia.[14] Women should be counseled in preventive measures, such as handwashing around young children and immunocompromised individuals.

Previously, rejection risk was considered higher during pregnancy, but further study indicates that this is not the case. The NTPR reported a rejection rate of 19% in 36 heart recipients in 2007 and a 21% rate in 33 patients in 2004, with many showing low-grade rejection that did not require further treatment and no maternal graft loss up to 2 years postpartum.[10,20]

Other pregnancy-related risks are similar to that in the general pregnant population, including hyperemesis gravidarum and deep venous thrombosis/pulmonary embolism.[11] Hyperemesis gravidarum presents the risk of subtherapeutic immunosuppression drug levels, which should be

monitored closely. Heart transplant recipients are already at risk for venous thromboembolism[21] and thus additional vigilance is required in pregnant heart transplant recipients with any symptoms or signs of deep venous thrombosis/pulmonary embolism.

Fetal risk includes a 15% to 20% rate of spontaneous abortion, a 2% stillbirth rate, and up to 33% with low birth weight.[20] There is a risk of premature delivery, primarily due to spontaneous preterm labor as well as to preeclampsia necessitating early delivery.

Intrapartum Management

A multidisciplinary team must craft a plan for delivery, including induction, mode of delivery, anesthesia, and extent of cardiac monitoring. Vaginal delivery is recommended with cesarean section reserved for obstetric indications; transplantation alone should not be the indication for cesarean section.[17] In the setting of significant graft dysfunction or clinical deterioration that could compromise maternal or fetal outcome, a multidisciplinary team of transplant cardiology, cardiac surgery, high-risk obstetrics, anesthesia, and neonatology determines if a scheduled cesarean section is the safest option.

Epidural anesthesia is considered well tolerated for pain control while also reducing the pain-induced sympathetic response and blood pressure fluctuations during labor.[14] Continuous electrocardiographic monitoring for arrhythmias is recommended during labor followed by serial electrocardiograms after delivery to monitor for ischemia. Central venous pressure or pulmonary artery pressure monitoring should be reserved for pregnant heart transplant recipients with significant graft dysfunction or pulmonary hypertension.[11] Antibiotic prophylaxis for delivery is indicated in transplant recipients with a history of infective endocarditis in the graft, significant valvulopathy (defined as regurgitation due to a structurally abnormal valve), and prosthetic valves or prosthetic material/residual patches used to repair cardiac lesions.[22] An uncomplicated cesarean section and vaginal delivery are not indications for antibiotic prophylaxis.[17]

Postdelivery Care and Maternal Complications

Immediately postdelivery, hemodynamic fluctuations begin with increases in cardiac output and stroke volume due to increased cardiac preload from autotransfusion of uteroplacental blood into the intravascular space.[14,23] Because the uterus decompresses after delivery, mechanical compression of the vena cava releases and further increases preload. Patients with normal graft function should tolerate these hemodynamic changes well. In the setting of graft dysfunction, however, women are most vulnerable to these hemodynamic alterations in the immediate postpartum period.

Barrier methods and combination hormonal contraception are acceptable forms of contraception in the transplant patient; hormonal contraception should be avoided for similar nontransplant indications (hypercoagulable states, hypertension, liver disease, and estrogen-sensitive cancers).[18]

Immunosuppression drug levels again require close monitoring as maternal intravascular volume and metabolism changes return to normal. Development of sensitization and HLA antibodies must be monitored in a transplant patient postpregnancy, the consequences of which are discussed later.

SENSITIZATION

Heart transplant recipients in the current era are more likely to be sensitized (ie, have preformed antibodies against HLA). Women are at higher risk for sensitization, and one of the major risk factors for sensitization is pregnancy. Other risk factors include transfusions, ventricular assist devices, and prior transplantation. Such preformed antibodies may cause hyperacute rejection, increase the risk of rejection after transplantation,[24] and

predispose patients to the development of cardiac allograft vasculopathy.[25]

Detection of Anti-human leukocyte antigens Antibodies

Currently, the detection of anti-HLA antibodies is most commonly performed using solid phase assays. With these assays, latex beads bound with single HLAs are mixed with patient serum. Antibodies bind to their respective antigen-coated beads, are tagged with an anti-IgG fluorescent carrier, and are then detected by flow cytometry. In this manner, the identity and quantification of anti-HLA antibodies are accomplished. Quantification is important, because antibodies of greater intensity in vitro are considered potentially more than cytotoxic in vivo. The presence of anti-HLA antibodies in high levels (usually median fluorescence intensity [MFI] above 5000) is considered potentially cytotoxic.[25]

Intensity of antibodies may not be the best test of potential cytotoxicity, however, because not all antibodies at high intensity may be detrimental to graft function. Because newer studies indicate the ability of donor-specific antibodies to fix complement, a functional assay may be a better marker of their cytotoxicity[26,27] Activation of the classical complement pathway by antibodies begins with their binding of C1q, the first component of the pathway. Once activated by C1q, the classical pathway leads to the formation of the membrane attack complex and ultimately results in cell lysis and death. Thus, antibodies with the ability to bind C1q are expected to be more likely cytotoxic, and this has been borne out in renal transplant recipients.[26,28] For centers where the C1q assay is not currently available, considering only antibodies that are strong binding by MFI after a 1:8 dilution may offer comparable information.[27]

Fig. 2 outlines an approach to the detection of anti-HLA antibodies in heart transplant candidates and how the presence of such antibodies would change management for patients awaiting transplantation.

Approach to the Crossmatch

The detection of anti-HLA antibodies prior to transplantation is important because donors are avoided who have HLA corresponding to high-level anti-HLA antibodies in a potential recipient, because this is a risk for hyperacute rejection. In the past, the only way to assess for this was with a prospective crossmatch, in which a potential recipient's serum was mixed with donor cells to assess for complement-dependent cytotoxicity. This severely geographically restricted the donor

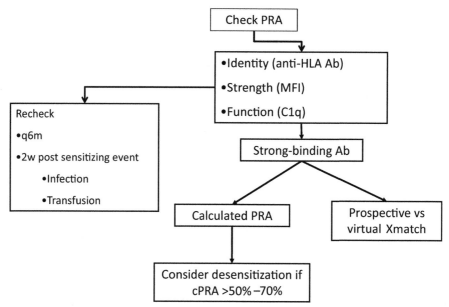

Fig. 2. Management of the sensitized heart transplant patient. Sensitized patients are those with a positive panel reactive antibody (PRA) screen. Ab, antibodies; Xmatch, crossmatch; The next step is to determine the identity and intensity of the anti-HLA antibodies. This information can be used for the virtual crossmatch and to determine the cPRA. If the cPRA is above 50% to 70%, desensitization therapy may be used. cPRA = frequencies of those antigens in the donor population. The cPRA computes the PRA percentage using both anti-HLA class I and class II antibody specificities, assigned to each patient as unacceptable, and knowledge of the frequency of the assigned unacceptable HLA antigens in a representative population. (*Adapted from* Kittleson MM, Kobashigawa JA. Antibody-mediated rejection. Curr Opin Organ Transplant 2012;17(5):522; with permission.)

pool to hospitals near where the candidate's serum was stored, however, thus reducing the number of potential donors for this patient.

The virtual crossmatch has replaced the prospective crossmatch at most centers. With the virtual crossmatch, HLA corresponding to high-level anti-HLA antibodies in the transplant candidate are listed as "avoids" in the United Network for Organ Sharing database; thus, potential donors with such HLA are not considered. This method has proved safe and successful in heart transplantation.[29]

Ultimately, however, the major decision is which HLA to avoid, and this is an art as well as a science. For those recipients with many high-level HLA antibodies, avoiding the HLA corresponding to the very highest intensity (or complement-biding) antibodies might be chosen, to allow for consideration of all potential donors. Choosing to avoid HLA corresponding to only the most potentially cytotoxic anti-HLA antibodies in the virtual crossmatch would broaden the donor pool, potentially at the expense of delayed hyperacute rejection; thus, this approach is often reserved only for unstable candidates unable to tolerate a long wait time to transplantation.

The Calculated Panel Reactive Antibody

The identity and intensity of anti-HLA antibodies are useful not only in safely finding a donor organ for a sensitized recipient but also in deciding which sensitized patients require treatment prior to transplantation.[24,25] Centers often use a threshold of the calculated panel reactive antibody (cPRA) to decide on treatment of a sensitized patient. The cPRA is the frequency of unacceptable HLA in the donor population.[30] cPRA highlights the fact that not all high-level anti-HLA antibodies are created equally, and some have an impact on the ability to find a suitable donor heart more than others.[31] As with deciding on which HLA to avoid when listing a patient for transplantation, deciding which HLA to include in the cPRA computation is an art as well as a science. The more antibodies that are included, the higher the cPRA. If the cPRA is above 50%, therapies to reduce antibody levels prior to transplantation may be used.

Approach to Desensitization

Management of the sensitized patients involves protocols to target antibodies by inactivation

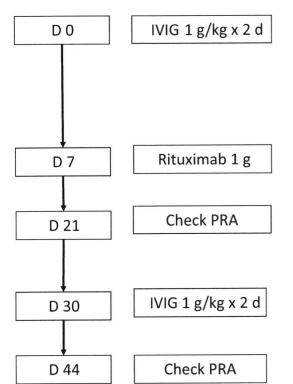

Fig. 3. Desensitization protocol for status 2 patients. The treatment of circulating antibodies depends on the cPRA. Treatment is considered for those patients with cPRA greater than 50% to 70%. For status 2 patients, desensitization using IVIG and rituximab typically is used. (*Reprinted from* Kittleson MM, Kobashigawa JA. Management of the highly sensitized patient awaiting heart transplant. Available at: https://www.acc.org/latest-in-cardiology/articles/2014/12/22/17/07/management-of-the-highly-sensitized-patient-awaiting-heart-transplant-expert-analysis. Accessed September 4, 2018; with permission.)

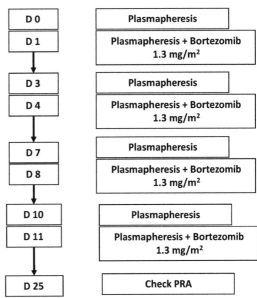

Fig. 4. Desensitization of status 1A patients or those with refractory antibodies. For status 1A patients awaiting transplantation, or those with refractory antibodies despite IVIG and rituximab, bortezomib is used. This regimen lowers antibodies more effectively in these patients. (*Reprinted from* Kittleson MM, Kobashigawa JA. Management of the highly sensitized patient awaiting heart transplant. Available at: https://www.acc.org/latest-in-cardiology/articles/2014/12/22/17/07/management-of-the-highly-sensitized-patient-awaiting-heart-transplant-expert-analysis. Accessed September 4, 2018; with permission.)

(intravenous immunoglobulin [IVIG],[32] removal (plasmapheresis), and decreased production [rituximab[32]] and bortezomib[33]). Production of IVIG begins with pooled human plasma from several thousand screened volunteer donors, from which highly purified polyvalent IgG is derived. Although the mechanisms of action are incompletely understood, IVIG suppresses inflammatory and immune-mediated processes. Rituximab is a monoclonal antibody directed against the CD20 antigen on B-lymphocytes. It is most commonly used for B-cell lymphoma but also, in conjunction with IVIG, reduces HLA antibodies in patients awaiting kidney transplantation (**Fig. 3**).[32]

If the protocol of IVIG and rituximab is ineffective in reducing the cPRA below 50%, or if a patient requires rapid desensitization (ie, listed status 1A), then bortezomib, a proteasome inhibitor against plasma cells, may be used (**Fig. 4**). It is most commonly used for the treatment of multiple myeloma but also reduces HLA antibodies in patients awaiting heart transplantation.[33] To increase effectiveness, bortezomib can be combined with plasmapheresis over a 2-week cycle with plasmapheresis on the day before and day of bortezomib administration (days 0, 1, 3, 4, 7, 8, 10, and 11).

Eculizumab

Pretransplant interventions with IVIG, rituximab, and bortezomib can reduce antibodies levels such that it is possible to find an acceptable donor. Hyperacute rejection at the time of transplantation related to preformed cytotoxic anti-HLA antibodies can still occur, however, due to donor-specific antibodies that were considered unlikely to be cytotoxic by virtual crossmatch or that formed after banked blood was collected for a prospective crossmatch. In this setting, eculizumab offers further insurance and protection against hyperacute rejection.

Eculizumab is a monoclonal antibody that selectively inhibits the terminal portion of the complement cascade. The complement cascade is activated by antigen-antibody complexes and ultimately leads to formation of the membrane attack complex, culminating in cell death. Eculizumab specifically binds to the terminal complement component 5 (C5) and ultimately prevents the generation of the terminal complement complex C5b-9. Eculizumab is Food and Drug Administration approved for use in paroxysmal nocturnal hemoglobunuria and atypical hemolytic-uremic syndrome, 2 complement-mediated conditions. Benefit has been seen, however, in sensitized kidney transplant recipients.[34]

SUMMARY

Heart transplantation is an established therapy for end-stage heart failure, and women comprise approximately half of all transplant recipients. Although women have superior post-transplant survival, they fare worse on some markers of health-related quality of life, and post-transplant coping strategies can be tailored accordingly. A frank discussion of the risks of pregnancy must be accomplished with female heart transplant recipients of childbearing age and specific treatment approaches may be implemented. Successful outcomes have been reported with the appropriate multidisciplinary team management beginning in the preconception period. Finally, women are more likely to be sensitized and recent advances in the management of sensitized heart transplant candidates may allow more women to safely undergo heart transplantation.

REFERENCES

1. Yancy CW, Jessup M, Bozkurt B, et al. 2013 ACCF/AHA guideline for the management of heart failure: a report of the American College of Cardiology Foundation/American Heart Association Task Force on Practice Guidelines. Circulation 2013;62(16):e147–239.

2. Lund LH, Khush KK, Cherikh WS, et al. The Registry of the International Society for Heart and Lung Transplantation: thirty-fourth Adult Heart Transplantation Report—2017; Focus Theme: allograft ischemic time. J Heart Lung Transplant 2017;36(10):1037–46.

3. Jalowiec A, Grady KL, White-Williams C. Gender and age differences in symptom distress and functional disability one year after heart transplant surgery. Heart Lung 2011;40(1):21–30.

4. Grady KL, Naftel DC, Young JB, et al. Patterns and predictors of physical functional disability at 5 to 10 years after heart transplantation. J Heart Lung Transplant 2007;26(11):1182–91.

5. Rybarczyk B, Grady KL, Naftel D, et al. Emotional adjustment five years after heart transplant: a multi-site study. Rehabil Psychol 2007;52:206–14.

6. White-Williams C, Wang E, Rybarczyk B, et al. Factors associated with work status at 5 and 10 years after heart transplantation. Clin Transplant 2011;25(6):E599–605.

7. Grady KL, Naftel DC, Kobashigawa J, et al. Patterns and predictors of quality of life at 5 to 10 years after heart transplantation. J Heart Lung Transplant 2007;26(5):535–43.

8. Grady KL, Andrei AC, Li Z, et al. Gender differences in appraisal of stress and coping 5 years after heart transplantation. Heart Lung 2016;45(1):41–7.

9. Lowenstein BR, Vain NW, Perrone SV, et al. Successful pregnancy and vaginal delivery after heart transplantation. Am J Obstet Gynecol 1988;158(3 Pt 1):589–90.

10. Armenti VT, Radomski JS, Moritz MJ, et al. Report from the National Transplantation Pregnancy Registry (NTPR): outcomes of pregnancy after transplantation. Clin Transplant 2004;103–14.

11. Abdalla M, Mancini DM. Management of pregnancy in the post-cardiac transplant patient. Semin Perinatol 2014;38(5):318–25.

12. O'Boyle PJ, Smith JD, Danskine AJ, et al. De novo HLA sensitization and antibody mediated rejection following pregnancy in a heart transplant recipient. Am J Transplant 2010;10(1):180–3.

13. Drenthen W, Pieper PG, Roos-Hesselink JW, et al. Outcome of pregnancy in women with congenital heart disease: a literature review. J Am Coll Cardiol 2007;49(24):2303–11.

14. Wu DW, Wilt J, Restaino S. Pregnancy after thoracic organ transplantation. Semin Perinatol 2007;31(6):354–62.

15. Rasmusson K, Brunisholz K, Budge D, et al. Peripartum cardiomyopathy: post-transplant outcomes from the United Network for Organ Sharing Database. J Heart Lung Transplant 2012;31(2):180–6.

16. Casale JP, Doligalski CT. Pharmacologic considerations for solid organ transplant recipients who become pregnant. Pharmacotherapy 2016;36(9):971–82.

17. McKay DB, Josephson MA, Armenti VT, et al. Reproduction and transplantation: report on the AST Consensus Conference on Reproductive Issues and Transplantation. Am J Transplant 2005;5(7):1592–9.

18. Costanzo MR, Costanzo MR, Dipchand A, et al. The International Society of Heart and Lung Transplantation Guidelines for the care of heart transplant recipients. J Heart Lung Transplant 2010;29(8):914–56.

19. Pisoni CN, D'Cruz DP. The safety of mycophenolate mofetil in pregnancy. Expert Opin Drug Saf 2008;7(3):219–22.

20. Ohler L, Coscia LA, McGrory CH, et al. National Transplantation Pregnancy Registry (NTPR): pregnancy outcomes in female thoracic transplant recipients. J Heart Lung Transplant 2007;26:S158.

21. Elboudwarej O, Patel JK, Liou F, et al. Risk of deep vein thrombosis and pulmonary embolism after heart transplantation: clinical outcomes comparing upper extremity deep vein thrombosis and lower extremity deep vein thrombosis. Clin Transplant 2015; 29(7):629–35.

22. Nishimura RA, Carabello BA, Faxon DP, et al. ACC/AHA 2008 guideline update on valvular heart disease: focused update on infective endocarditis: a report of the American College of Cardiology/American Heart Association Task Force on Practice Guidelines endorsed by the Society of Cardiovascular Anesthesiologists, Society for Cardiovascular Angiography and Interventions, and Society of Thoracic Surgeons. J Am Coll Cardiol 2008;52(8): 676–85.

23. Gandhi M, Martin SR. Cardiac disease in pregnancy. Obstet Gynecol Clin North Am 2015;42(2):315–33.

24. Kobashigawa J, Mehra M, West L, et al. Report from a consensus conference on the sensitized patient awaiting heart transplantation. J Heart Lung Transplant 2009;28(3):213–25.

25. Kobashigawa J, Crespo-Leiro MG, Ensminger SM, et al. Report from a consensus conference on antibody-mediated rejection in heart transplantation. J Heart Lung Transplant 2011;30(3):252–69.

26. Loupy A, Lefaucheur C, Vernerey D, et al. Complement-binding anti-HLA antibodies and kidney-allograft survival. N Engl J Med 2013;369(13): 1215–26.

27. Zeevi A, Lunz J, Feingold B, et al. Persistent strong anti-HLA antibody at high titer is complement binding and associated with increased risk of antibody-mediated rejection in heart transplant recipients. J Heart Lung Transplant 2013;32(1):98–105.

28. Sutherland SM, Chen G, Sequeira FA, et al. Complement-fixing donor-specific antibodies identified by a novel C1q assay are associated with allograft loss. Pediatr Transplant 2012;16(1):12–7.

29. Stehlik J, Islam N, Hurst D, et al. Utility of virtual crossmatch in sensitized patients awaiting heart transplantation. J Heart Lung Transplant 2009; 28(11):1129–34.

30. Cecka JM. Calculated PRA (CPRA): the new measure of sensitization for transplant candidates. Am J Transplant 2010;10(1):26–9.

31. Cecka JM, Kucheryavaya AY, Reinsmoen NL, et al. Calculated PRA: initial results show benefits for sensitized patients and a reduction in positive crossmatches. Am J Transplant 2011;11(4):719–24.

32. Vo AA, Lukovsky M, Toyoda M, et al. Rituximab and intravenous immune globulin for desensitization during renal transplantation. N Engl J Med 2008;359(3): 242–51.

33. Patel J, Everly M, Chang D, et al. Reduction of alloantibodies via proteosome inhibition in cardiac transplantation. J Heart Lung Transplant 2011;30(12):1320–6.

34. Stegall MD, Diwan T, Raghavaiah S, et al. Terminal complement inhibition decreases antibody-mediated rejection in sensitized renal transplant recipients. Am J Transplant 2011;11(11):2405–13.

Pulmonary Hypertension in Women

Veronica Franco, MD, MSPH[a],*, John J. Ryan, MD[b], Vallerie V. McLaughlin, MD[c]

KEYWORDS

- Pulmonary hypertension • Pulmonary arterial hypertension • Women • Pregnancy

KEY POINTS

- The prevalence of pulmonary arterial hypertension (PAH) is higher in women.
- The prognosis is overall better for female compared with male patients with PAH.
- Pregnancy is associated with significant risk, mortality, and morbidity in patients with PAH; consensus guidelines recommend against pregnancy and counsel about early termination in these patients.
- Recent advances in treatment showed some improvement in prognosis in small case reports of pregnant patients with PAH, particularly with the early use of parental prostacyclin starting around 30 weeks.
- Education is fundamental for women with PAH of childbearing age for pregnancy prevention as well as discussion about birth control methods.

INTRODUCTION

Pulmonary hypertension (PH) can be caused by a wide range of medical conditions and is separated into groups depending on cause. Group 1 PH or pulmonary arterial hypertension (PAH) is uncommon and characterized by an angioproliferative vasculopathy of the distal pulmonary circulation. PH secondary to left-sided heart disease is referred to as group 2 PH. Heart failure with preserved ejection fraction is one of the most common causes of group 2 PH and is predominantly in women, as long-standing comorbidities like hypertension and diabetes are common in older women. Group 3 PH is PH secondary to chronic hypoxic lung disease. Group 4 PH is a rare condition referred to as chronic thromboembolic PH (CTEPH), and group 5 PH is a mix of miscellaneous diseases (**Box 1**).[1]

PAH is predominantly a disease of women with a ratio of 2:1 in the United Kingdom and Ireland[2] and French registries[3] and 4:1 in the US Registry to EValuate Early And Long-term Pulmonary Arterial Hypertension Disease Management (REVEAL).[4] Female to male prevalence varies depending on ethnicity; the ratio is 3.2:1 in the white population, 4.7:1 in the Hispanic population, 5.5:1 in the black population, and 3.9:1 in other races, such as Native American, Pacific Islander, Asian, or other/unknown.[5] The prognosis is better in women

Disclosure: V. Franco has served on advisory boards for Gilead, Bayer, and United Therapeutics. The Ohio State University has received research funding from Actelion Pharmaceuticals, ARENA, REATA, Bayer, Gilead, and United Therapeutics. V.V. McLaughlin has served as a consultant and/or advisor for Actelion Pharmaceuticals US, Inc, Bayer, Merck, St. Jude Medical, and United Therapeutics Corporation. The University of Michigan has received research funding from Actelion Pharmaceuticals US, Inc, Arena, Bayer, and Sonovie. J.J. Ryan has no disclosures.
[a] Division of Cardiovascular Medicine, Department of Medicine, The Ohio State University, 473 W 12th Avenue, DHLRI Suite 200, Columbus, Ohio 43210, USA; [b] Division of Cardiovascular Medicine, Department of Medicine, University of Utah, Salt Lake City, UT, USA; [c] Division of Cardiovascular Medicine, Department of Medicine, University of Michigan, Ann Arbor, MI, USA
* Corresponding author.
E-mail address: Veronica.Franco@osumc.edu

Heart Failure Clin 15 (2019) 137–145
https://doi.org/10.1016/j.hfc.2018.08.013
1551-7136/19/© 2018 Elsevier Inc. All rights reserved.

Box 1
Comprehensive clinical classification of pulmonary hypertension

PAH (1)

Idiopathic

Heritable

  $BMPR_2$ mutation

  Other mutations

Drugs and toxins

Associated with

  Connective tissue disease

  HIV infection

  Portal hypertension

  Congenital heart disease

  Schistosomiasis

1′ Pulmonary venoocclusive disease

1′ Pulmonary capillary hemangiomatosis

1″ Persistent PH of the newborn

PH due to left heart disease (2)

HF with reduced ejection fraction

HF with preserved ejection fraction

Valvular disease

Congenital heart disease/acquired

  Pulmonary vein stenosis

  Left heart inflow/outflow obstruction

  Cardiomyopathies

PH due to lung disease/hypoxia (3)

Chronic obstructive pulmonary disease

Interstitial lung disease

Mixed restrictive and obstructive disease

Sleep breathing disorder

Chronic exposure to high altitude

Developmental lung disease

Chronic thromboembolic/obstructions (4)

CTEPH

Other pulmonary artery obstructions

  Angiosarcoma

  Other intravascular tumors

  Arteritis

  Congenital pulmonary artery stenosis

  Parasites (hydatidosis)

PH of unclear/multifactorial mechanism (5)

Hematological disorders

Chronic hemolytic anemia

Myeloproliferative disorders

Splenectomy

Systemic disorders

  Sarcoidosis

  Pulmonary histiocytosis

  Lymphangioleiomyomatosis

  Neurofibromatosis

Metabolic disorders

  Glycogen storage disease

  Gaucher disease

  Thyroid disease

Others

  Tumoral thrombotic microangiopathy

  Fibrosing mediastinitis

  Chronic renal failure (w or w/o dialysis)

  Segmental PH

Abbreviations: $BMPR_2$, bone morphogenetic protein receptor type 2; HF, heart failure; HIV, human immunodeficiency virus; w, with; w/o, without.

Adapted from Simonneau G, Gatzoulis MA, Adatia I, et al. Updated clinical classification of pulmonary hypertension. J Am Coll Cardiol 2013;62(25, Supp. D):D36; with permission.

with PAH compared with male patients,[6] with the 5-year survival from diagnosis of PAH being estimated at 62% in women compared with 52% in men.[7]

The focus of this article is on group 1 PH, exploring the pathophysiology behind the differences in incidence and survival and also detailing clinical scenarios in PH that are unique to women, specifically pregnancy.

PULMONARY ARTERIAL HYPERTENSION

Defined by a resting hemodynamics of mean pulmonary artery pressure (mPAP) of 25 mm Hg or greater, wedge pressure of 15 mm Hg or less, and pulmonary vascular resistance (PVR) of greater than 3 woods units; significant cardiac, pulmonary, or thromboembolic diseases have to be excluded.[1] The upper level of normal for resting mPAP is 20 mm Hg, and it is unclear how to classify and manage patients with mPAP of 21 to 24 mm Hg. Most of the relevant epidemiologic and therapeutic studies in PAH have used the 25-mm Hg threshold.

Idiopathic PAH (iPAH) accounts for approximately half of the cases of PAH, whereby no identifiable cause is found.[4] Hereditary transmission has been reported in up to 10% of patients, and three-quarters of hereditary cases of PAH have been linked to bone morphogenetic protein receptor type 2 mutations.[8] Drug- and toxin-induced PAH has been described with methamphetamines, anorexigens, L-tryptophan, and rapeseed oil.[1] Dasatinib, a tyrosine kinase inhibitor used for hematologic malignancies, has also been linked with PAH.[9] PAH associated with connective tissue disorders are almost 25% of all cases. The prevalence of PAH in scleroderma is 8% to 12% and is associated with significant morbidity and mortality.[10] Human immunodeficiency virus–related PAH incidence is independent of the CD_4 cell count. Portopulmonary hypertension occurs in about 5% of the patients with portal hypertension and increases mortality perioperatively during liver transplantation if the mPAP is greater than 35 mm Hg.[11]

ROLE OF ESTROGEN IN PULMONARY ARTERIAL HYPERTENSION

It remains unclear as to why a female predominance exists in PAH, although there are several theories. Lower testosterone levels in female patients may make the pulmonary vasculature and right ventricle (RV) more vulnerable to insults.[12] Testosterone acts as a pulmonary vasodilator through calcium antagonism not through classic androgen receptor signaling.[13] Dehydroepiandrosterone is an important mediator of the female predominance, as it is produced at the highest level and attenuates hypoxic vasoconstriction. It has been shown to be protected against the development of PH in male rat models.[14,15] Estrogen has vasodilatory properties and mediates these effects through α and β receptors using a nitric oxide–dependent mechanism.[16] Small changes in plasma estrogen levels can have major consequences on vascular function and physiologic fluctuations in estrogen, such as is seen with menstruation, and can reduce pulmonary artery constrictor responses.[17]

CLINICAL CHARACTERISTICS AND RESPONSE TO THERAPY

As previously mentioned, the prognosis of PAH in women is better than that observed in men. Analysis of patient-level data from 6 randomized controlled trials of endothelin receptor antagonists (ERAs) identified sex and race differences in response to ERAs. After 12 weeks of therapy, placebo-adjusted 6-minute walk distance improved by 16.7 m in men versus 44.1 m in women.[18] Some

of these differences could originate from estrogen effects in the RV. A sex difference in RV function has been also observed in registry data. Men without cardiovascular disease have a lower RV ejection fraction (RVEF) compared with women,[19] and higher estradiol levels are associated with higher RVEF in women using hormone therapy.[20]

Five-year survival was worse in male patients at 63% compared with female patients with 85%, in a retrospective review despite no difference in therapy between males and females. Importantly, men were not noted to be sicker at baseline, as neither the right heart catheterization hemodynamics at baseline, nor at follow-up, showed significant differences between men and women. However, men had worse functional class, shorter 6-minute walk distances, and higher brain natriuretic peptide (BNP) levels at follow-up compared with female patients.[21] One possible explanation for the observed outcome difference could be the change in RV function: RVEF improved by 3.6% in women with the initiation of PAH-specific therapies but decreased by 1.0% in men. Approximately 30% of the effect of sex on survival was accounted for by the differences in RVEF at follow-up.

PREGNANCY AND PULMONARY ARTERIAL HYPERTENSION

Pregnancy poses a vast risk to women with PAH.[1,22] The European Society of Cardiology (ESC)/European Respiratory Society's (ERS) 2015 guidelines for the diagnosis and treatment of PH,[1] the ESC's guidelines on cardiovascular disease in pregnancy,[23] and the Pulmonary Vascular Research Institute's (PVRI) statement in pregnancy[24] state that pregnancy in women with PAH should be avoided and all patients should be counseled about therapeutic early termination. The pregnancy-associated mortality rate remains high in the prostacyclin era, but there is a higher rate of survival in recent case series.[25–28]

The third trimester and first month after delivery represent the period of highest risk for patients with PAH, and mortality is driven by the development of refractory severe RV failure, pulmonary thrombosis, or pulmonary hypertensive crisis (Fig. 1).[23–33] Elevated pulmonary pressures associated with right heart failure and the use of general anesthesia were independent risk factors for mortality. Immediately post partum, PVR increases and RV contractility may subsequently decrease. Hypotension can also occur because of blood loss or vasovagal response to pain. These changes, in the face of a drop in preload, set the stage for cardiovascular collapse in patients with PAH. Sudden death may also occur from

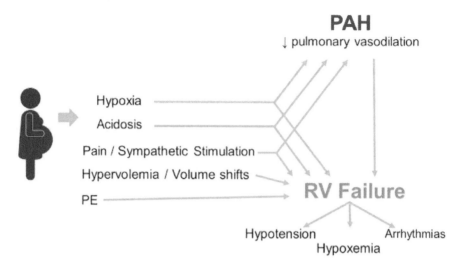

Fig. 1. Pathophysiology of right ventricular (RV) failure in pregnant patients with PAH. PE, pulmonary embolism. (*Data from* Elwing JM, Panos RJ. Pregnancy and pulmonary arterial hypertension. In: Sulica R, Preston I, editors. Pulmonary hypertension-from bench research to clinical challenges. Rijeka (Croatia): InTech; 2011. p. 289–304.)

numerous other mechanisms, including pulmonary embolism, arrhythmias, or stroke from intracardiac shunts.

A meta-analysis of reported cases in the National Library of Health (MEDLINE) between 1978 and 1996,[29] the preprostacyclin era, showed that maternal mortality rates of 36% in Eisenmenger syndrome, 30% in primary PH (now called iPAH), and 56% in PH associated with other conditions (secondary vascular PH), P<.08 versus the other 2 groups. In this study, all fatalities occurred within 35 days after delivery, except for 3 prepartum deaths due to Eisenmenger syndrome. Neonatal survival ranging from 87% to 89% was similar in the 3 groups. Maternal mortality independent risk factors included late diagnosis (P = .002, odds ratio 5.4) and late hospital admission (P = .01, odds ratio 1.1 per week of pregnancy).

Epoprostenol was approved by the Food and Drug Administration (FDA) in 1995 and other 11 specific PAH vasodilators have been used since 2001. Four databases have been published with the use of prostacyclins during pregnancy[25–28] (**Table 1**):

1. Outcomes in 26 women: Sixteen pregnancies were successful, and healthy babies without complications were delivered.[25] Three women (12%) died and one (4%) developed RV failure requiring urgent heart-lung transplantation. Calcium channel blocker responders and women with near-normal hemodynamics had favorable outcomes. All patients who died had severe uncontrolled PAH with PVR close to 20 wu. Neonatal mortality was 12%.

2. Outcomes in 18 cases: Twelve women continued the pregnancy.[26] Most patients underwent catheterization (66%) at the time of hospital admission; all required hospitalization at 29 ±1.4 weeks for worsening dyspnea (12 of 12), dizziness (9 of 12), chest pressure (5 of 12), and/or syncope (3 of 12). Six patients were on parental prostacyclins initially, and 2 more were started at approximately 25 to 29 weeks. Cesarean delivery was performed in all patients at a median of 34 weeks using epidural (n = 8) or general anesthesia (n = 3). One patient died at the time of diagnosis at 29 weeks of pregnancy and one died 6 weeks post partum due to sepsis. No fetal deaths occurred.

3. Outcomes in 5 pregnancies: All had good outcomes for both mothers and neonates.[27] Patients were systematically evaluated by a multidisciplinary group of PAH specialists, cardiologists, maternal-fetal medicine, and obstetrics anesthesiology; every case was discussed on a monthly basis. All patients were treated with low-molecular-weight heparin and started on intravenous (IV) prostacyclins at approximately 30 weeks. Patients were admitted 1 week before the planned delivery. Vaginal delivery with assisted second stage was the preferred route of delivery. Invasive peripartum monitoring with an arterial line and a goal central venous pressure (CVP) of 10 to 12 mm Hg to maintain an adequate preload were used. All patients were discharged on IV prostacyclin; oral PAH therapy was started approximately

Table 1
Pregnancy in patients with pulmonary arterial hypertension: case reports

Study	Preg	Timing	Centers No.	PAH Classification	Mortality	Need for Transplant	Good Outcomes	PAH Therapy
Weiss[29]	125	1978–1996	n/a	Idiopathic, congenital associated PAH	30% 36% 56%	2 (<1%)	n/a	None
Jais[25]	26	2007–2010	13 (United States, Eur, Aus)	Idiopathic, congenital associated PAH	3 (12%)	1 (4%)	62% preg	CaCB (31%) IV/SQ prost (23%)
Duarte[26]	6	1999–2009	5 (United States)	Idiopathic, congenital associated (CTD)	2 (17%)	0	83% preg	IV/SQ prost (67%) PDE-5i (33%)
Smth[27]	5	n/a	1 (United States)	Idiopathic, congenital associated (CTD)	0%	1 (Transplant ill advised)	100% preg	IV prost (100%) PDE-5i (40%)
Bedart[28]	73	1997–2007	n/a	Idiopathic, congenital associated PAH	17% 28% 33%	n/a	n/a	CaCB (26%) IV/SQ prost (41%) PDE-5i (7%) ERA (3%)

Abbreviations: Aus, Australia; CaCB, calcium channel blockers; CTD, connective tissue disease; ERA, endothelin receptor antagonist; Eur, Europe; IV, intravenous; n/a, not available; PDE-5i, phosphodiesterase 5 inhibitor; preg, pregnancies; prost, prostacyclin; SQ, subcutaneous.

2 months post partum with the goal to wean prostacyclin.

4. Outcomes of 47 cases series and reports in the National Library of Health (MEDLINE) between 1997 and 2007,[28] which included 73 pregnant patients with PAH: More than two-thirds of the deaths occurred within the first month after delivery. Maternal mortality was overall significantly lower compared with the previous era[29] (25% vs 38%, $P = .047$). The lower maternal mortality may be related to an earlier diagnosis with prompt referral to an experienced PH center and initiation of PAH therapy, particularly IV prostacyclins. Yet, there were 3 fetal deaths (10%) and neonatal morbidity was significant with 90% preterm deliveries.

Monitoring During Pregnancy

Recommendations for the management of pregnant women with PAH have been published recently.[23,24,30] Referral to an expert PAH center is fundamental, where patients will be followed closely by a multidisciplinary group, including collaboration of PH specialists, obstetricians, critical care specialists, and neonatologists[23,24,30–32]; a plan of care should be detailed early on, including timing for specific PAH therapy initiation and time and mode of delivery for the baby.

During pregnancy, patients need to be evaluated at least every 4 weeks in the first 2 trimesters and more frequently in the third trimester.[23,24,30,31] BNP and supplemental oxygen is recommended to maintain oxygen saturation greater than 90%. Echocardiography on a regular basis is recommended for maternal RV function monitoring and frequent ultrasounds for the fetus to evaluate growth. With improved maternal outcomes in the prostacyclin era, there seems to be significantly more morbidity in the neonates, with a higher proportion of premature deliveries (85% vs 59% in iPAH and 86% vs 53% in PAH associated with congenital disease).[28,29] Hospitalization of women with PAH in the late second or early third trimester is sometimes appropriate because of the increased risk of premature labor and of hemodynamic complications.[31,34]

Continuous Swan-Ganz monitoring utility remains uncertain.[23,24,29] However, CVP of approximately 10 to 12 mm Hg may be very beneficial at the time of delivery[27,31] to assure appropriate preload and volume status,[27] whereas a CVP greater than 15 mm Hg should raise concern for decompensated RV failure and prompt for RV support therapy like diuresis or inotropes. Close blood pressure monitoring and a fast treatment of hypotension with fluids or pressors is fundamental, particularly at the time of delivery and in the immediate postpartum period.[31,34]

Evaluation for lung transplantation should be performed in a timely manner. The effects of pregnancy on the cardiovascular system may persist for several months after delivery[35]; late deaths were reported at 14, 19, and 24 months post partum. It remains unclear if the cause of death was due to the pregnancy itself or progression of PAH. Nonetheless, emphasize the importance of close follow-up after delivery up to 2 years.

PAH Therapy During Pregnancy

Endothelin receptor blockers and riociguat are contraindicated because of the teratogenic effects (category X). Prostanoids and phosphodiesterase 5 inhibitors (PDE-5i) are classified as a risk category B and have not been associated with fetal abnormalities. Iloprost has been shown to be associated with adverse fetal effects in animals (risk category C) but has been used successfully without adverse human fetal effects in a series of 9 patients.[33]

Background therapy with calcium channel blockers, prostanoids, and PDE-5i should be continued during pregnancy. The initiation of calcium channel blockers in patients not known to be responsive is contraindicated.[1] Parental prostacyclins are potent vasodilator of both the pulmonary and systemic circulation and considered to be the drug of choice during pregnancy,[25–28] and the best outcomes were obtained when they were initiated early in the third trimester. The ERS and PVRI guidelines[1,23,24] do not recommend one specific therapeutic regimen but recommend close monitoring of the pregnant PAH patient, continuation of background therapy and a low threshold to initiate parental prostacyclins in the late second or early third trimesters. If prostacyclins are initiated, they should be continued for at least a few months post partum to assure hemodynamic stability.

Anticoagulation During Pregnancy

There is a 4- to 10-fold increase in venous thrombosis during pregnancy. Microparticles shed from the cell membranes of maternal endothelial cells and platelets are also associated with enhanced thrombosis.[33] Acute pulmonary embolism in women with PAH, with an already deranged pulmonary vasculature, can precipitate significant RV failure.

Anticoagulation has been used in most case studies.[24–28] Guidelines[23] recommend that in patients whereby the indication for anticoagulation outside pregnancy is established, anticoagulation should also be maintained during pregnancy. In PAH associated with congenital cardiac shunts in the absence of significant hemoptysis, anticoagulant treatment should be considered in patients with pulmonary artery thrombosis or signs of heart failure.

Vitamin K antagonists are contraindicated in the first trimester because of their teratogenic risk for fetal craniofacial abnormalities and can lead to fetal hemorrhage and spontaneous abortion at any stage of pregnancy. The use of any anticoagulation potentially can increase the risk of bleeding, particularly at delivery and early post partum. Anticoagulation risks and benefits should be assessed on an individual basis and may not be well tolerated in select patient groups, such as those with Eisenmenger syndrome or other bleeding diathesis. Anticoagulation could be considered for patients with PAH.[23,24,30–34] If anticoagulation will be used, most recommend the use of low-molecular-weight heparin during pregnancy to transition to prophylactic dosing before delivery and then resumed with oral anticoagulants after delivery if there is no contraindication.

Mode of Delivery

The optimal timing and mode of delivery for pregnant women with PAH have not been determined, but women with PAH should ideally not go into labor naturally.[23,30] Practices vary across centers, with successful vaginal births (using induction and assisted delivery) and cesarean deliveries. Epidural is the preferred method of anesthesia. Patients receiving general anesthesia have a 4-fold increase in mortality.[28]

Emergency deliveries are associated with higher mortality rates. Spontaneous vaginal delivery can potentially lead to labor at night or during weekends with inexperienced teams managing the labor and delivery. Vaginal birth is usually associated with less blood loss, fewer infections, less thromboembolic risk, and less abrupt hemodynamic changes compared with a cesarean delivery. However, prolonged labor can be detrimental and can produce hypercarbia, acidosis, and hypoxia. Pain and Valsalva maneuvers can increase myocardial oxygen consumption. If vaginal delivery is selected, it should be performed in the intensive care unit or the operating room. Use of forceps during delivery may shorten the second stage of labor and be associated with a lower mortality rate, particularly in patients with Eisenmenger syndrome.[27,31]

Scheduled cesarean delivery can be performed in a more controlled environment, with close multidisciplinary management and extracorporeal membrane oxygenation on standby as needed. Even though it is associated with anesthesia risk, this will avoid a lengthy labor, particularly a prolonged second stage and the need to bear down. Planned cesarean deliveries are usually arranged for 32 to 37 weeks of pregnancy. Most importantly, regardless of the modes of delivery, is that the underlying PAH treatment is optimized.

BIRTH CONTROL IN PULMONARY ARTERIAL HYPERTENSION

Education is fundamental for women with PAH of childbearing age for pregnancy prevention as well as discussion about methods of birth control.[1,31] There is no consensus related to the most appropriate method of birth control.[1,24,31] Barrier methods, such as condoms, coils, and intrauterine devices, are safe and could be considered for temporary prevention. Permanent measures, like tubal ligation, are alternatives; but invasive procedures may be complicated by vasovagal syncope with the placement of the device and/or pain during and after the procedure. Sometimes a combination of 2 methods is recommended.

Pharmacologic therapies are adequate methods of birth control for women with PAH. Progesterone is not associated with an increased risk of thrombosis and may be the most appropriate birth control method, and progesterone-only contraceptives are beneficial. There is some controversy regarding the use of medroxyprogesterone acetate (Depo-Provera), given the thromboembolic risk; but the risk may not be as high with concomitant warfarin. However, progesterone may interact with warfarin; close anticoagulation monitoring is recommended. Estrogen formulations may increase the risk of venous thromboembolism, but lower-dose preparations with concurrent anticoagulation are a reasonable option. It is important to mention that bosentan, an ERA, can decrease the efficacy of pharmacologic therapies; the utilization of 2 methods is recommended for patients using this therapy.

HORMONE REPLACEMENT THERAPY IN PULMONARY ARTERIAL HYPERTENSION

It is unclear whether the use of hormonal therapy in postmenopausal women with PAH is advisable. It may be considered in cases of intolerable menopausal symptoms in conjunction with oral anticoagulation.[1]

SUMMARY

The prevalence of PAH is higher in women, and the reason for this remains unclear. Prognosis is overall better for female compared with male patients with PAH, likely because of the favorable effects of estrogen in RV function. Current treatment guidelines advise to avoid pregnancy for patients with PAH because of the significant risk, particularly in the postpartum time, which is associated with high mortality and morbidity for both mothers and neonates. Recent advances in treatment showed improvement in prognosis in small case report series, particularly with the early use of parental prostacyclin starting approximately 30 weeks; yet, there has not been a large database published with pregnancy outcomes.

REFERENCES

1. Galiè N, Humbert M, Vachiery JL, et al. 2015 ESC/ERS guidelines for the diagnosis and treatment of pulmonary hypertension: The Joint Task Force for the Diagnosis and Treatment of Pulmonary Hypertension of the European Society of Cardiology (ESC) and the European Respiratory Society (ERS): endorsed by: Association for European Paediatric and Congenital Cardiology (AEPC), International Society for Heart and Lung Transplantation (ISHLT). Eur Heart J 2016;37:67–119.

2. Ling Y, Johnson MK, Kiely DG, et al. Changing demographics, epidemiology, and survival of incident pulmonary arterial hypertension: results from the pulmonary hypertension registry of the United Kingdom and Ireland. Am J Respir Crit Care Med 2012;186:790–6.

3. Humbert M, Sitbon O, Chaouat A, et al. Pulmonary arterial hypertension in France: results from a national registry. Am J Respir Crit Care Med 2006; 173:1023–30.

4. Badesch DB, Raskob GE, Elliott CG, et al. Pulmonary arterial hypertension: baseline characteristics from the REVEAL registry. Chest 2010;137:376–87.

5. Frost AE, Badesch DB, Barst RJ, et al. The changing picture of patients with pulmonary arterial hypertension in the United States: how REVEAL differs from historic and non-US Contemporary Registries. Chest 2011;139:128–37.

6. Humbert M, Sitbon O, Chaouat A, et al. Survival in patients with idiopathic, familial, and anorexigen-associated pulmonary arterial hypertension in the modern management era. Circulation 2010;122:156–63.

7. Shapiro S, Traiger GL, Turner M, et al. Sex differences in the diagnosis, treatment, and outcome of patients with pulmonary arterial hypertension enrolled in the registry to evaluate early and long-term pulmonary arterial hypertension disease management. Chest 2012;141:363–73.

8. Machado RD, Pauciulo MW, Thomson JR, et al. BMPR2 haploinsufficiency as the inherited molecular mechanism for primary pulmonary hypertension. Am J Hum Genet 2001;68:92–102.

9. Guignabert C, Phan C, Seferian A, et al. Dasatinib induces lung vascular toxicity and predisposes to pulmonary hypertension. J Clin Invest 2016;126:3207–18.

10. Gall H, Felix JF, Schneck FK, et al. The giessen pulmonary hypertension registry: survival in pulmonary hypertension subgroups. J Heart Lung Transplant 2017;36:957–67.

11. Swanson KL, Wiesner RH, Nyberg SL, et al. Survival in portopulmonary hypertension: Mayo Clinic experience categorized by treatment subgroups. Am J Transplant 2008;8:2445–53.

12. Pugh ME, Hemnes AR. Pulmonary hypertension in women. Expert Rev Cardiovasc Ther 2010;8:1549–58.

13. Jones RD, English KM, Pugh PJ, et al. Pulmonary vasodilatory action of testosterone: evidence of a calcium antagonistic action. J Cardiovasc Pharmacol 2002;39:814–23.

14. Farrukh IS, Peng W, Orlinska U, et al. Effect of dehydroepiandrosterone on hypoxic pulmonary vasoconstriction: a $Ca(2+)$-activated $K(+)$-channel opener. Am J Physiol 1998;274:L186–95.

15. Oka M, Karoor V, Homma N, et al. Dehydroepiandrosterone upregulates soluble guanylate cyclase and inhibits hypoxic pulmonary hypertension. Cardiovasc Res 2007;74:377–87.

16. Lahm T, Crisostomo PR, Markel TA, et al. Selective estrogen receptor-alpha and estrogen receptor-beta agonists rapidly decrease pulmonary artery vasoconstriction by a nitric oxide-dependent mechanism. Am J Physiol Regul Integr Comp Physiol 2008;295:R1486–93.

17. Lahm T, Patel KM, Crisostomo PR, et al. Endogenous estrogen attenuates pulmonary artery vasoreactivity and acute hypoxic pulmonary vasoconstriction: the effects of sex and menstrual cycle. Am J Physiol Endocrinol Metab 2007;293:E865–71.

18. Gabler NB, French B, Strom BL, et al. Race and sex differences in response to endothelin receptor antagonists for pulmonary arterial hypertension. Chest 2012;141:20–6.

19. Kawut SM, Lima JA, Barr RG, et al. Sex and race differences in right ventricular structure and function: the multi-ethnic study of atherosclerosis-right ventricle study. Circulation 2011;123:2542–51.

20. Ventetuolo CE, Ouyang P, Bluemke DA, et al. Sex hormones are associated with right ventricular structure and function: the MESA-right ventricle study. Am J Respir Crit Care Med 2011;183:659–67.

21. Jacobs W, van de Veerdonk MC, Trip P, et al. The right ventricle explains sex differences in survival in idiopathic pulmonary arterial hypertension. Chest 2014;145:1230–6.

22. McLaughlin VV, Archer SL, Badesch DB, et al. ACCF/AHA 2009 expert consensus document on pulmonary hypertension. Circulation 2009;119:2250–94.

23. Regitz-Zagrosek V, Lundqvist CB, Borghi C, et al. ESC guidelines on the management of cardiovascular diseases during pregnancy. Eur Heart J 2011;32: 3147–97.

24. Hemnes AR, Kiely DG, Cockrill BA, et al. Statement on pregnancy in pulmonary hypertension from the Pulmonary Vascular Research Institute. Pulm Circ 2015;5:435–65.

25. Jäis X, Olsson KM, Barbera JA, et al. Pregnancy outcomes in pulmonary arterial hypertension in the modern management era. Eur Respir J 2012;40: 881–5.

26. Duarte AG, Thomas S, Safdar Z, et al. Management of pulmonary arterial hypertension during pregnancy: a retrospective, multicenter experience. Chest 2013;143:1330–6.

27. Smith JS, Mueller J, Daniels CJ. Pulmonary arterial hypertension in the setting of pregnancy: a case series and standard treatment approach. Lung 2012; 190:155–60.

28. Bedard E, Dimopoulos K, Gatzoulis MA. Has there been any progress made on pregnancy outcomes among women with pulmonary arterial hypertension? Eur Heart J 2009;30:256–65.

29. Weiss BM, Zemp L, Seifert B, et al. Outcome of pulmonary vascular disease in pregnancy: a systematic overview from 1978 through 1996. J Am Coll Cardiol 1998;31:1650–7.

30. Olsson KM, Channick R. Pregnancy in pulmonary arterial hypertension. Eur Respir Rev 2016;25: 361–3.

31. Hsu CH, Gomberg-Maitland M, Glassner C, et al. The management of pregnancy and pregnancy-related medical conditions in pulmonary arterial hypertension patients. Int J Clin Pract Suppl 2011; 175:6–14.

32. Olsson KM, Jais X. Birth control and pregnancy management in pulmonary hypertension. Semin Respir Crit Care Med 2013;34:681–8.

33. Elwing JM, Panos RJ. Pregnancy and pulmonary arterial hypertension. In: Sulica R, Preston I, editors. Pulmonary hypertension-from bench research to clinical challenges. Rijeka (Croatia): InTech; 2011. p. 289–304.

34. Warnes CA. Pregnancy and pulmonary hypertension. Int J Cardiol 2004;97:11–3.

35. Clapp JF III, Capeless E. Cardiovascular function before, during, and after the first and subsequent pregnancies. Am J Cardiol 1997;80:1469–73.

Printed and bound by CPI Group (UK) Ltd, Croydon, CR0 4YY

03/10/2024

01040385-0010